SPORTS MEDICINE
FOR PARENTS & COACHES

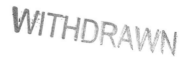

SPORTS
MEDICINE
FOR PARENTS & COACHES

DANIEL J. BOYLE, M.D.

GEORGETOWN UNIVERSITY PRESS

WASHINGTON, D.C.

Georgetown University Press, Washington, D.C.
© 1999 by Georgetown University Press. All rights reserved.
Printed in the United States of America
10 9 8 7 6 5 4 3 2 1   1999
This volume is printed on acid-free offset book paper.

Library of Congress Cataloging-in-Publication Data

Boyle, Daniel J.
    Sports medicine for parents and coaches /
    Daniel J. Boyle.
            p.   cm.
    ISBN 0-87840-732-4 cloth. — ISBN 0-87840-733-2 paper
            1. Pediatric sports medicine—Handbooks, manuals, etc.
    2. Sports injuries in children—Handbooks, manuals, etc.
    I. Title.
    RC1218.C45B69 1999
    617.1'027'083—dc21

                                                        99-13392
                                                        CIP

CONTENTS

FOREWORD

When someone writes a book, particularly if the author is employed full time during the writing process, many people other than the author deserve credit for the accomplishment. I would like to acknowledge some of the people who made this publication possible. First, my wife Margie, who struck the perfect balance between prodding and encouraging me when I hit those inevitable stumbling blocks known as writer's block. I would like to thank my twelve children: Justin, Elizabeth, Jude, Eammon, Kathleen, Daniel, Aloysius, Bridget, Charlie, Mary, Molly, and Rose. It was through attending their thousands of sporting events as they grew up that I conceived of the idea for this book and from which I gleaned most of my clinical insights. Mary Rakow, a neighbor and good friend, made the first attempt to edit this manuscript. She demonstrated to me how much I had forgotten about sentence structure and how often I lapsed into passive voice. Ed Egan, another good friend, encouraged me to begin this project at a time when I wasn't sure that I was adding anything important to the existing literature on the subject. Ed is the father of eight athletes and is also a coach, so if he thought a book like this was needed, then I guess it was. Mark Murphy, the athletic director at Colgate University and an All-Pro defensive back for the Washington Redskins, and Joseph Caroso, M.D., team physician for the Pittsburgh Pirates, were each kind enough to review the manuscript. JoAnn Robinson, my office manager, and Erin Vitale, my medical assistant, helped me keep me in contact with the publishers for the last-minute changes. The staff at Georgetown University Press, particularly John Samples, Gail Grella, Ivan Osorio, and Deborah Weiner, showed enormous patience in dealing with a "rookie" author. I also thank medical illustrators David Klemm, Peter Y. Stone, and Michele Prosise for preparing the final drawings. To these people and many others I owe a lot for all that is good about this book. Any errors are mine alone.

Daniel J. Boyle, M.D.
June 1, 1999

PREFACE

I remember sitting at a T-ball game watching a father who was about twenty years younger than I. His son, who was a good athlete, had just fielded a ground ball at shortstop. The batter was running to first base. Instead of throwing the batter out, the shortstop ran across the diamond in an attempt to tag the runner out. Of course, the runner was safe at first base, and the father was exasperated. He expected his son to catch a ground ball coming off a bat and turn and throw in a totally different direction to get the player out at first base. The boy was a six-year-old, and this was his very first T-ball game. Six-year-olds are just beginning to develop both the learning skills and the motor skills to accomplish these two very different and difficult tasks—fielding a batted ball and throwing to a base—but the father expected his son to perform like Cal Ripkin!

I'm the father of twelve children aged twenty-seven to nine. I've been around sports for most of my life and I am a physician with a special certification in sports medicine. Because of my background and training, I just *knew* that the boy would catch the ball and run at the batter. I was amazed that the father of the boy didn't know it as well. Then I realized that parents aren't born with an innate knowledge of developmental pediatrics; they can't be expected to know when their children are ready and able to perform certain complicated tasks that sports participation requires.

That same year I watched a very talented athlete pitch in several Little League games. He started the season brilliantly, but his talent seemed to abandon him as the season neared its end. I asked the coach the cause of the boy's failures, and he told me that "his arm was dead." I examined the pitcher and found that he had shoulder instability caused by overpitching. As I took a history, I found out that the player was so good that he pitched on three different baseball teams in different leagues at the same time. It was obvious that he was suffering from an overuse injury of his shoulder. I advised the pitcher to stop throwing for the rest of the season and prescribed exercises over the winter to strengthen the shoulder. The next year the athlete came back and had an "all star" season, limiting his pitching to one team in one league and playing shortstop on the other teams.

At first I thought that my common sense had helped save the boy's playing career, and I wondered how the parents and coaches could have been so irresponsible as to let the player pitch too often. But the more that I thought about it, the more I realized that it was medical knowledge, not common sense, that had benefited the child. Parents and coaches are not always aware of the causes of illnesses and injuries that affect young athletes, and they don't necessarily know how to treat these injuries. Since I do know about these things, I decided to write this book to share my insights with coaches and parents whose children are participating in sports.

I began to be interested in sports medicine before it became a formal discipline. I stood on the sidelines at my children's games and took care of athletes who suffered injuries. After a while parents sought me out because they knew that I had a special interest in youth sports problems.

Sports medicine was once the province of orthopedic surgery. Now that medicine is more complex, the field of sports medicine is, too. It includes medical problems involving the nervous, cardiovascular, digestive, and genitourinary systems as well as the skin. These problems are beyond the scope of orthopedics. Today there is a great deal of interest in sports medicine among many different medical specialties. The boards of family practice, internal medicine, pediatrics, and emergency medicine have begun to award certificates of added qualification in sports medicine to acknowledge that some of their members have special training and expertise in this field. The members of these primary care specialty boards realize that the family physician or pediatrician is often better equipped to deal with the breadth of sports medicine issues than is the orthopedic surgeon.

These primary care doctors are today's sports medicine experts. They are familiar with heart murmurs that would exclude a youth from participation in high school basketball. They are expert at counseling the athlete about the risk of transmitting HIV through sports contacts and the treatment of dermatological conditions that may limit sports participation. These doctors have also seen their fair share of musculoskeletal injuries. The most important thing that these primary care sports medicine doctors bring to the table is that they are also expert in *preventing injuries*.

As a board-certified family physician with a certificate of added qualification in sports medicine, a team physician, a father of twelve children, and a coach, I wrote this book to share my expertise and experiences in sports medicine with you, the parents and coaches of youth athletes.

ONE

Preparing

Children

for Sports

Participation

INTRODUCTION

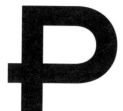articipation in sports is valuable for children, not only for its physical benefits but because it builds character and promotes social skills and concepts such as teamwork. Playing sports imposes structure and a set routine on children. It also requires and encourages a sense of commitment and instills an interest in achieving excellence. Participating in team and individual sports is a great confidence builder and teaches children how to deal with adversity. They also learn how to win graciously and to lose without shame, knowing that they did their best. Competing in athletics may further serve to divert children from involvement in crime, drugs and alcohol, and sex.

To help children take fullest advantage of all the benefits sports can offer, it is important for parents and coaches to make sure that the athletes start out and remain in good physical condition. This means dealing effectively with injuries and with health problems that may affect sports participation, either by preventing them in the first place or by treating them swiftly and prudently after they occur.

What do you do when your daughter comes home limping after a basketball game? Can your son wrestle if he has asthma? Your daughter, who is an excellent gymnast, had back pain in each of the last two years just as the state championship was about to begin. How can this disaster be avoided this year? These and countless other questions have been asked by parents about their children's participation in sports. They are all dealt with in this handy reference. This is a handbook. It is not meant to be encyclopedic but rather is intended to give the reader a general introduction to the topic.

This book covers the common injuries that young people suffer in sports competition and how to prevent or treat them. It deals with your child's physical and psychological development so that you, the parent, will know when your child is ready for a particular sport. It can be used as a reassuring reference when your child suffers a minor injury. I have paid particular attention to the injuries that are most dangerous as well as to those that seem minor at first but can cause long-term problems. This book tells you how to treat minor athletic injuries yourselves. It will help you understand how the sports medicine physician approaches your child's injuries.

This handbook is divided into five parts. Part 1 deals with preparing children for sports participation. Part 2 discusses the factors that go into maintaining good physical condition. Part 3 covers the treatment of specific injuries by anatomical location, and part 4 lists injuries that commonly occur in each sport and how to treat them. Part 5 describes the essential equipment to be included in a sports physician's medical bag (for the convenience of physician readers who might someday serve as doctors for their children's teams). The book concludes with a set of summary guidelines for the parents of young athletes.

In this era of managed care, a thorough explanation from the doctor is not often available to patients or their parents. This disappearing aspect of the art of medicine is particularly important when it involves the care of our children. This handbook will help fill that gap. It fleshes out the information that you get from your health care providers and may increase your sense of comfort that your child's injuries are getting the care and attention that they deserve.

Growth and Development of the Young Athlete

One of the questions that parents of young children most often ask is, "When can my child begin to play sports?" To answer this it is important to understand the basic facts of growth and development.

GENERAL GROWTH GUIDELINES

From age two to puberty, children grow two to three inches per year. Girls then undergo a pubertal growth spurt during which they grow approximately ten inches. Boys grow about eleven inches during their pubertal growth spurt.

Preschool

Infants and toddlers under the age of two have very poorly developed motor skills. At this age learning is also poorly developed, and thus repetitive practice of a skill is of no value. These children simply won't be able to do tomorrow what you taught them today. In addition, most children at this age are extremely far-sighted, which means that organized sports are beyond their ability. The eyeball is very flat at birth but gradually assumes a more rounded shape. By the time a child is six years old, the eye has achieved its adult shape and a child's vision is like an adult's.

The older preschooler, from age two to five, can run, throw, catch, and hop. Practice is still of little value for these three- and four-year-olds because of their extremely short attention span. Children at this age cannot grasp the concept of interacting with other children in sport, such as catching a batted ball and throwing to a base to get the runner out. Therefore, team sports are inappropriate at this age. Children aged three to five can swim, tumble, and play catch, but activities like ballet, T-ball, and gymnastics are not suitable for kids in this age group.

Ages Six to Nine

The six- to nine-year-old can begin to play team sports. By this time the child has begun to develop a sense of balance. The eye has developed its adult shape, and the farsightedness of the preschooler has disappeared; the child can follow a baseball or soccer ball in flight. Children at this age are beginning to learn how to interact with one another and to perceive spatial relationships. It is dawning on the young soccer player that she doesn't have to play the whole field but should stay in position and cover the area assigned to her. Appropriate individual sports for this age group are competitive swimming, tennis, and gymnastics. Good team sports are soccer or baseball. The players will have no trouble fielding the batted ball and throwing to a base, but they still lack the spatial skills necessary for more complicated plays.

DON'T IMPOSE YOUR ADULT UNDERSTANDING OF THE SPORT ON A NINE-YEAR-OLD.

This is a very difficult time for parents and coaches. It is a period of transition because some of the players are beginning to understand the concept of a complicated play, such as fielding a bunt, but many of their teammates are still clueless. Be patient. Apply the KIS principle: "Keep it simple." Don't try to instruct your young athletes to execute complex plays, and don't expect them to have enough of an attention span to stay focused on the game at all times. Don't impose your adult understanding of the sport on a nine-year-old. Be instructive and positive. Correct but don't criticize mistakes. Coaches often try to teach young players by repeating the same instructions over and over, but they will get better results if they demonstrate the drill and then *walk*, rather than *talk*, the players through it.

Ages Ten to Twelve

Ten- to twelve-year-olds can play games that we adults can also relate to. Children are able to play soccer and baseball competently and can begin to tackle more complex sports such as football, basketball, and wrestling. Many parents are reluctant to allow their ten-year-olds to play youth football, because they are afraid that their child may sustain a serious injury. However, in youth football the children are matched by both age and weight. For example, a nine-year-old can play on the ninety-five-pound team if he weighs no more than ninety-five pounds. A ten-year-old couldn't play on the same team unless he weighed ninety pounds or less, and an eleven-year-old would have to weigh eighty-five pounds or less to compete on the team. Through this combination of weight and age, the players are evenly matched. They are also all prepubertal. They don't have the muscle mass or the speed to severely injure one another. I have not seen a serious injury in youth football in the fifteen years that I have been associated with it.

Ages Thirteen to Fifteen

By the ages of thirteen to fifteen, children have the motor skills to play any sport at an adult level. They also have the learning skills to master complex basketball defenses and run stunts as football defensive linemen. The problem is that some of these athletes are postpubertal and some of them are still prepubertal. It doesn't take much imagination to understand what happens when the 180-pound postpubertal linebacker tackles the 90-pound prepubertal running back twenty-five times in a high school freshman football game. The solution is as elusive as the problem is simple. We can choose either the distasteful alternative of refusing to allow the smaller, less mature individual to go up against the more mature player, or the dangerous option of allowing him to compete. This dilemma is one that affects boys almost exclusively. Most girls have reached puberty by age fourteen, but puberty for boys may be extended to age sixteen. Additionally, this is a problem that is most obvious in the contact and collision sports—e.g., ice hockey, lacrosse, and football—which are more in the domain of males than females and where combatants are matched only by age, not by weight as they are in youth football. In these situations the understanding of the parents, coaches, and athletic directors is essential.

If the parents or the child's older siblings experienced delayed puberty, the child will probably do the same. If your child goes through puberty late and he's dying to play football, be consoled that the vast physiological differences that exist at age thirteen are all but erased by age eighteen, when everyone is, at least, two years postpubertal. Though going through puberty later than his or her peers is disconcerting at the time, there is a silver lining. These children are more likely to be taller by age eighteen than those who go through puberty earlier.

Tanner Stages of Development

In sports medicine we use Tanner stages to evaluate the development of boys and girls as they go through puberty. Suzanne Tanner, a sports medicine pediatrician, developed this system for looking at adolescents according to their degree of sexual development rather than their chronological age. Tanner stage 1 reflects prepubertal status and Tanner stage 5 reflects adult status. The intermediate Tanner stages cover the transition between these two extremes. By using Tanner stages, we can account for physical maturity as well as age when we help young athletes choose a sport in which they can compete successfully.

CHOOSING THE RIGHT SPORT

How can parents and coaches determine which sport is most appropriate for a particular child? In addition to having a general understanding of the growth process, it is important to consider the size and build of the individual child. In general, children can be expected to resemble their parents when it comes to body types: short parents have short kids; slightly built parents have small-framed ones. A small child will probably be happier choosing a sport that doesn't require height and brawn.

Another factor to consider is the child's age in relation to that of his classmates. If the cutoff age in your area for entering school is based on a January first birth date and your son was born in December, he will be eleven months younger than some of the children he will be competing against and will therefore also probably be smaller.

Ideally, parents and coaches should be able to avoid a situation in which a child ends up choosing a sport for which he or she is not physically suited. For example, a boy with a small frame and light weight should be directed toward soccer, baseball, or wrestling rather than football. On the other hand, if he has his heart set on playing high school football, don't burst his bubble. It can be rewarding for both boys and girls just to be part of a team, even if they are of small stature or have limited abilities.

If the child is an average athlete and wants to play on a team, it is a good idea to direct him or her to sports in which there are a large number of competitors. For example, the football team often has sixty or more participants, of whom about thirty-five will play in the typical game, whereas basketball and baseball teams have only fifteen to twenty players. Thus, if a boy learns the skills

TABLE 1. CONTACT AND NONCONTACT SPORTS

CONTACT		NONCONTACT		
CONTACT/ COLLISION	LIMITED CONTACT/ IMPACT	STRENUOUS	MODERATELY STRENUOUS	NONSTRENUOUS
Boxing	Baseball	Aerobic dancing	Badminton	Archery
Field hockey	Basketball	Crew	Curling	Golf
Football	Bicycling	Fencing	Table tennis	Riflery
Ice hockey	Diving	Field		
Lacrosse	Field	Discus		
Martial arts	High jump	Javelin		
Rodeo	Pole vault	Shot put		
Rugby	Gymnastics	Running		
Soccer	Horseback riding	Swimming		
Wrestling	Skating	Tennis		
	Ice	Track		
	Roller	Weight lifting		
	Skiing			
	Cross-country			
	Downhill			
	Water			
	Softball			
	Squash, handball			
	Volleyball			

needed for football when he is ten years old, he will probably be able to make the football team throughout high school. This principle applies to girls as well. Field hockey, soccer, and lacrosse have more competitors than some other sports and are thus more suitable for athletes of average ability. Both boys and girls should begin participating in their chosen sports at an early age so that they can make up in technique what they lack in physical skill.

The American Academy of Pediatrics has categorized a variety of sports according to the degree of contact and strenuousness of the effort involved (Table 1). A youth who is not able to compete in one type of activity may be able to play a different sport without limitation.

The Preparticipation Physical Examination

Over six million youth athletes are examined annually for medical clearance for sports participation. Children between the ages of two and eighteen should have physical exams yearly. Ideally, young athletes, especially those of high school age, should be examined by a pediatrician or family physician with an interest in and knowledge of sports medicine. A child participating in interscholastic high school sports will bring home a physical exam form with a series of medical history questions to be answered by the parents. (See pp. 110–111.) This information contained in the Evaluation is very important. Questions such as "Has anyone in your family died of heart problems or suddenly before the age of fifty?" are critically important. A "yes" answer to a question like this will prompt the physician to perform a particularly thorough cardiovascular exam that could lead to finding and treating a potentially life-threatening problem in a young athlete. Similarly, questions about asthma attacks, bee sting allergies, or previous injuries deserve your careful attention.

If the child does not bring the form home, he or she often fills it out hurriedly in the waiting or examination room at the doctor's office. One study published on this subject showed that parents and children give vastly different answers to medical questions. Parents should fill out the forms themselves. The task is too important to entrust to teenagers.

If you have a high school-aged son or daughter who plays sports, you may be aware that there are *two different types of preparticipation physical exams.* The first is the station exam, conducted in many high schools, in which large numbers of athletes move from station to station having their blood pressure recorded at one place, their orthopedic exam done at another, and so forth. This type of exam has the advantage of screening many children in a short time. The physicians involved are usually team physicians with an interest and expertise in sports medicine, and the exams are typically done at little or no cost to the student athletes.

The second type of exam is the physical done in your private physician's office. This type of exam has the advantage of being conducted one on one by a doctor who knows your child. This environment facilitates questions that the patient may be embarrassed to ask of a stranger in less private circumstances. The ideal situation is to have the exam done in a private office by a primary care physician with an interest in sports medicine.

Regardless of which type of exam you choose, the vast majority of children will pass. Only about one percent of children are disqualified from participating in their desired sport as a result of the preparticipation physical examination. Five to ten percent of the athletes tested require further evaluation and additional tests before they can be cleared to participate in sports.

In trying to decide whom to clear for sports participation, the sports medicine physician considers several issues. Will participation with a physical problem cause the athlete to risk injury to herself or someone else? Will participation cause an existing injury to get worse? Can we minimize these risks with treatment? If not, can the child participate in his sport in a limited way? For example, the starting centerfielder with rotator cuff tendinitis in his throwing arm can't play the outfield but can be a designated hitter or pinch runner until his injury heals. If the answers to all these questions disqualify the athlete, can we find another sport for this child?

Whichever type of exam you choose, you shouldn't wait until the week before practice begins to schedule the physical. The preparticipation examination should be conducted six to twelve weeks before the start of practice. This will allow time to correct any problem that is found or to perform special tests if indicated.

The most important consideration for parents of young athletes is to choose a physician who knows enough about sports medicine to ask the appropriate questions during the exam. Approximately two-thirds of the problems that our youth athletes have are identified while the doctor is taking the medical history (this is why it is so important for the parents to fill out the history questionnaires). The preparticipation physical examination, even when performed by a sports medicine primary care physician, should not be a terribly expensive proposition. All that is necessary in most cases are a history and physical examination. Special tests such as blood tests and x-rays are usually not indicated. In fact, several studies demonstrate that laboratory tests and x-rays are of no value in clearing healthy young athletes for sports participation.

Physical Conditions That Limit Sports Participation

What physical conditions prevent or limit participation in sports? The most obvious but certainly not the most serious physical impairment is the *absence of a paired organ,* such as an eye, kidney, or testicle. A boy missing one testicle should avoid full-contact and collision sports and should wear a plastic protective cup while playing limited contact sports such as basketball or baseball. An athlete who has only one kidney should avoid contact and collision sports. Even though the likelihood of a serious injury to the existing kidney is small, the consequences are dire if the organ is damaged. An athlete missing one eye should wear protective goggles made of polycarbonate, a shatterproof material, when playing racquet sports and basketball. When playing football, lacrosse, or ice hockey, he or she should wear an eye shield incorporated into the helmet, and an eye shield on the batting helmet is essential during baseball games and practice. Children with a significant visual impairment should be treated as if they were actually missing an eye. Anyone who has 20/50 corrected vision or worse in either eye should protect his or her eyesight as mentioned above. Ultimately, however, it is up to the athlete and parents to decide whether he or she plays. As parents and coaches, be responsible and reasonable in determining what forms of protection are in the child's best interests.

Less obvious but more serious are problems related to the cardiovascular system. These heart problems are responsible for the majority of deaths among young athletes. One of the leading causes of death is *congenital heart disease,* an abnormal heart anatomy that a child is born with. Some types of heart disease cannot be detected because the children don't show any symptoms. Unfortunately, these are first diagnosed at the time of a serious cardiac event. Those that can be detected often manifest themselves by the presence of a heart murmur. Any youth athlete over the age of eight whose doctor finds a murmur on the preparticipation exam, even if he or she believes that the murmur is an innocent one, should get an echocardiogram.

There are many physical conditions that require temporary restrictions for participation in certain sports, such as poorly controlled diabetes, high blood pressure, or seizures. The athlete may resume participation when these conditions are under control. Players shouldn't practice or play strenuous sports when they have an acute illness associated with a fever or after suffering a concussion. Infectious mononucleosis is another temporary contraindication to participation in sports where contact is possible. This restriction applies to sports such as diving or baseball as well as the traditional contact or collision sports. In mononucleosis the spleen, an organ located on the upper left side of the abdomen, enlarges and is susceptible to rupture. I typically keep athletes out of competition in contact and collision sports for four weeks from the time of diagnosis, even if there is no evidence of spleen enlargement. If the spleen is enlarged on examination, I prevent the athlete from competing until there is evidence of a normal spleen by ultrasound exam. This may take several months.

Certain issues unique to female athletes should also be addressed during the preparticipation physical exam. I advise teens to wear a sports bra during training and competition to lessen the incidence of breast injury. The bra should provide adequate support and stabilization of the breasts during running. It can be purchased at most sporting goods and department stores.

I also ask questions about the athletes' menstrual cycles to find out whether the girls have started their periods and if so, whether they are menstruating regularly. Osteoporosis, a disease associated with older women, occurs with alarming frequency among teenage female athletes who are not having regular periods. Regular menstrual cycles range from twenty-four to thirty-five days in length. A girl who has begun menstruating will usually settle into a pattern of regular menses. If she has fewer than four menstrual cycles per year, she is at high risk for osteoporosis and should see her physician.

More than two million Americans with medical disabilities compete in some type of athletic event. Twelve percent of school-aged children are physically challenged. The parents of a physically challenged child should understand that their child has the same potential to reap the rewards from competition and team play as his or her able-bodied counterparts. Because they must overcome greater difficulties, participation in sports may bring even more satisfaction to athletes with physical disabilities than to those who are not similarly affected. It also gives them a way to vent their frustration with their condition in a socially acceptable way.

Blind athletes compete in skiing, weightlifting, and track and field. They are tethered to a sighted companion who leads the way while skiing or running. *Deaf athletes* compete in the same sports as blind athletes. Additionally, they can compete against able-bodied athletes in sports such as baseball and basketball. I once served as a team physician at a football game where one entire team was composed of deaf students competing against a school team composed of hearing students. One of the deaf students would beat a large bass drum on the sidelines to indicate that a receiver should begin in motion. A second drumbeat would indicate when the ball should be snapped. When the student beat the drum, players on the field could feel the reverberations in the ground and thus knew when to react. *Children confined to wheelchairs* compete in skiing, basketball, and tennis. There are leagues in most major metropolitan areas for wheelchair athletes.

Physically challenged athletes suffer an injury rate that is similar to that of their able-bodied counterparts. The types of injuries that they sustain, like strains, sprains, and contusions, are also the same. However, there are a few injuries that are unique to handicapped participants.

Wheelchair-bound children have an increased incidence of upper-extremity injuries because they use their upper limbs to propel themselves. There are also more abrasions and lacerations as a result of collisions with other wheelchair participants. Paraplegic children have no use of their legs. Quadriplegic athletes have lost function of their upper as well as lower extremities. Quadriplegics and paraplegics in wheelchairs suffer from pressure sores and are at risk for lower-extremity fractures because disuse of their lower extremities has led to osteoporosis. Properly padded chairs go a long way to cut down on these types of injuries. These athletes also have an increased rate of bladder problems. Because of their paralysis, they can't sense when their bladders are full, and the bladders can become overdistended. Therefore, these athletes are at risk of bladder rupture as a consequence of contact. They should make certain to empty their bladders before competition. They also have an extremely difficult time with regulation of their body temperatures because they can't sweat. The injury to the spinal cord that caused their paralysis affects the nerves that control sweating.

Many children with mild to moderate *asthma* compete successfully in several sports. They often need to inhale bronchodilators about twenty minutes before their event so that they can compete without symptoms. An asthma attack is more likely to occur while the athlete is competing in cold weather or during the spring or fall when the child is susceptible to pollen-related symptoms such as itchy eyes, sneezing, or a runny nose. Parents of severely asthmatic children might need to select a sport for them that is less likely to trigger an asthma attack, such as swimming. For a winter sport, basketball makes more sense than cross-country skiing, although asthmatics have won Olympic medals in cross-country skiing. Water sports are particularly well suited for the asthmatic patient because they breathe warm, humidified air, and the air immediately about the surface of the water is moist and warm.

Diabetics, like asthmatics, can successfully compete in any sport. The most common problem of the diabetic athlete is hypoglycemia, or low blood sugar, during practice or competition. Hypoglycemia can be prevented by altering the timing or dosage of the insulin injection before competing. Diabetic children usually use an insulin pump or take multiple doses of a short-acting insulin, and they can measure their own blood glucose levels with a glucometer or similar device that makes adjusting the dosage even easier. Sometimes the diabetic athlete misjudges his or her insulin needs before competition. If the athlete takes too much insulin, the blood sugar may drop to dangerously low levels, causing hypoglycemia. When this happens diabetics will become shaky, agitated, confused, irrational, and even combative because they aren't getting enough sugar to the brain to make it function properly. If a diabetic does have a *hypoglycemic attack,* he or she should immediately be given something to increase blood sugar.

Traditionally, orange juice with extra sugar added has been the treatment of choice. I prefer a tube of icing used for cake decorating, which is almost pure sugar. I always carry a tube of it in my medical bag when I attend sporting events as a team physician.

I have cared for many children who have *attention deficit disorder* (including a couple of my own children). Though this problem is not anywhere near as severe a disability as being blind or paraplegic, it is a disability that sometimes requires treatment during practice and competition. If these children require medication for school, they will often benefit from medication while participating in sports. Children who are taking Ritalin, Cylert, or Dexedrine for their attention deficit disorder should take these medications before games and practices. Medical studies have demonstrated that these children perform much better athletically as well as academically when they take their medication.

TWO

Maintaining Good Physical Condition

CONDITIONING

PRESEASON TRAINING

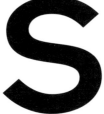

Statistically, school-age athletes suffer many more injuries during fall sports than in either winter or spring sports. The obvious explanation is that football is played during the fall. There are many injuries in football because it is a collision sport and because there are a large number of partici-pants. There is, however, another reason. More injuries occur in the fall because the students come back to school in September out of shape. Poorly conditioned athletes are injured more frequently than those who are in shape. Once the academic and sports year has started, a student may participate in cross-country running, then basketball, then field hockey. The first sport serves as a conditioning program for the later sports. As noted earlier, preparticipation exams should be conducted six to twelve weeks before the season begins, and so should a conditioning program. The youth soccer coach does not expect his players to show up at the first practice in shape to play, but the high school freshman soccer coach does! The preseason conditioning should start at least six weeks before the first practice so that the partici-pant is able to jog for forty-five minutes by the time practice begins.

WEIGHT TRAINING

Strength is required for most sports. I recommend that postpuber-tal boys participate in a weight-training program three days per week during the six-week conditioning period before their season begins. Prepubertal males and both pre- and postpubertal females, however, gain little strength by lifting weights. The male sex hormone, testosterone, is the chemical in the body that enables us to gain muscle mass and strength. Both boys and girls produce a small amount of testosterone in their adrenal glands, but most of this hormone is produced in the male testicles once puberty has begun. After puberty males gain significant strength by engaging in a weight-training program.

Many people, including some physicians, refuse to let their sons lift weights as young teenagers. This notion is not based on scien-tific evidence, but rather it stems from the fact that teenage boys sustain injuries lifting weights because they do not lift properly. In the past young boys were encouraged to lift heavy weights to prepare for their sports. They measured their progress by seeing how much weight they could lift at one time. This is a very ill-advised practice because it leads to a large number of injuries.

To build strength, boys should lift heavy weights several times. I tell them to work with a weight that they can lift five times. They are instructed to do three to five sets of five repetitions, resting three minutes between sets. Once they can perform this routine comfortably, I suggest that they increase to six, then seven repetitions, and finally to eight. Once they can do eight repetitions, I recommend that they increase the weight and go back down to five reps and build up again. Body builders who want bulk rather than strength should do more repetitions with lighter weights. There are very few teens who are lifting for bulk or muscle definition.

TO BUILD STRENGTH, BOYS SHOULD LIFT HEAVY WEIGHTS SEVERAL TIMES.

If athletes want endurance, they should use even lighter weights for more repetitions, perhaps fifteen to twenty "reps." Weight lifting should be done three or four times per week. It is simpler to exercise all muscles three times a week but makes more sense to exercise four days a week on the following schedule: flexor muscles (those that bend a joint) on Monday and Thursday and extensor muscles (those that straighten a joint) on Tuesday and Friday. In either case, I recommend that the athlete perform three to five sets of each exercise in each exercise session, with a three-minute break between sets.

HEAT AND HUMIDITY

Fall sports begin in the heat of August, and heat-related injuries are more likely to occur in unconditioned athletes of any age. In youth sports heat is even more of a problem for two reasons. First, youth athletes are more likely than their older counterparts to be out of shape. Second, because they are smaller than adults, youngsters don't dissipate heat as well. As adults, we also know to drink fluids liberally; kids have to be reminded.

Teams should not practice when temperature and humidity are high. Almost two hundred heat-related deaths occur annually in this country, and some of them occur among youth football players. Football coaches and athletic directors should be familiar with the wet-bulb temperature, which measures the combined effect of heat and humidity. When it exceeds eighty-five degrees, practice competition should be canceled. Your team doesn't have to buy a lot of expensive equipment to monitor heat and humidity. Local weather stations give a "humiture" reading based on this index.

And while we are talking about the weather, remember that thunderstorms, which occur often in the fall and spring, can be dangerous because of the accompanying lightning. Don't let children practice during a thunderstorm!

Vigorous physical activity causes us to lose over five pounds as a result of sweating for each hour that we exercise. Coaches should weigh players before and after practices and make sure they gain back the fluid weight lost during practice over the next twenty-four hours. Five and one-half pounds of weight lost from sweating requires about two and one-half quarts of fluids replacement. About one-half of these fluids should be replaced during the four hours immediately after practice, with the remainder being replaced during the rest of the day. Athletes who practice and play in hot weather should consume fluid until their urine is clear. Yellow urine means that the athlete is relatively dehydrated. Parents should take particular note of this; it is an important concept for you to understand when your sons and daughters are exercising vigorously in the heat. You may not be able to rattle off wet-bulb temperatures, but you can ask your children if their urine is clear or yellow.

On particularly hot days our football team will hold two short practice sessions rather than one long one: one in the early morning and one in the late afternoon to minimize heat-related illness. Many high school football leagues have rules that players practice the first week without wearing pads to facilitate heat acclimation without the burden of heavy clothing that inhibits heat dissipation.

Our bodies gradually become acclimated to exercise in the heat. It takes approximately two weeks for the players to become used to practicing and playing in the heat. During this time it is particularly important to warn our children about symptoms of heat exhaustion: fatigue, nausea, muscle cramps, and light-headedness. An athlete should immediately stop practice if any of these symptoms occur. You should send your child to practice well hydrated by having him or her drink a glass or two of water or one of the commercial sports drinks, such as Gatorade, before practice. Do not let your child drink iced tea or soft drinks that contain caffeine, which make us lose fluids and can make dehydration worse. Coaches should schedule water breaks every twenty to thirty minutes to make sure that the children are drinking enough. There is much debate as to which drink is best. A drink containing 5 percent carbohydrate (e.g., Gatorade) is absorbed slightly faster than water and is therefore preferred.

! Tips for coaches:

The idea that drinking fluids during practice causes cramping is a myth. The kids need the fluids. When I was playing youth sports we took salt tablets to replace the salt lost as a result of sweating. Salt tablets can cause gastrointestinal problems and should be avoided. We get enough salt in the average diet to replace our losses.

Once a child suffers heat exhaustion, he or she is more susceptible to a second episode; therefore, watch these athletes particularly closely. African-American children with sickle-cell trait are particularly susceptible to heat-related problems (see the section on sickle-cell disease, p. 22).

WARMING UP AND COOLING DOWN

When I began playing youth sports in the mid-fifties, I was told that warming up before exercise helped to prevent injuries. Coaches today preach the same thing. It would be very unusual to see a practice or a game in any sport without the obligatory pregame conditioning. Despite this long and venerable tradition, there are no data to show that warming up before exercise helps prevent injuries. I am convinced, however, that it does.

We can conveniently divide the pregame warm-up into two categories: general exercises and sport-specific exercises. If we take a baseball pitcher as an example, jogging around the outfield before the game would be a general exercise and throwing in the bull pen would be sport-specific. The general exercises often include calisthenic stretching exercises. These exercises can be static, where we stretch and hold our position for ten or fifteen seconds, or ballistic, where we bounce at the end of our stretch to extend the muscle farther. Everyone associated with sports medicine in the 1990s now knows that the ballistic stretch injures the muscle by causing a reflex contraction and should not be practiced.

Though there may be no data to support the benefit of pregame stretching, I believe that there is an advantage to pregame calisthenics in youth sports. Young children need something to help them make the mental transition from one activity to another. The warm-up helps to focus their attention on the game at hand. Even for older youth athletes the warm-up is important because it helps them mentally prepare for competition. It is part of the ritual of sport. When you stand on the sidelines at a high school football game and watch the athletes go through their pregame warm-ups, you can feel the excitement and intensity building among the participants.

! Tips for coaches:

Passive stretching, in which one member of a team stretches a teammate's muscle, should not be done. When we actively stretch our muscles, we stop at the point of discomfort. When we are passively stretched by a teammate, we can be pulled too forcefully and injury results. Just about every football team that I've seen on any level violates this recommendation. When I watch the pregame calisthenics, I see one player stretch another's arm, leg, or neck. I also invariably see a player injured this way because he was too macho to tell the other player to stop when he was being stretched to the point of pain.

IT IS MORE BENEFICIAL TO STRETCH MUSCLES ALREADY WARM FROM EXERCISE BECAUSE THEY STRETCH FARTHER WITHOUT INJURY.

What about cooling down after exercise? The time immediately after exercise is an ideal time to stretch. It is more beneficial to stretch muscles already warm from exercise because they stretch farther without injury. Stretching after aerobic exercise, such as track and cross-country, helps promote flexibility. If we go back to the example of the baseball pitcher mentioned earlier, it would be preferable for him to jog in the outfield and then do his calisthenics. I would also recommend stretching the muscles one at a time. This promotes maximum muscle lengthening. If your left hamstring is tight because of an old injury and you stretch both hamstring muscles together, the right hamstring is not being stretched very much. Certain stretching exercises isolate each muscle so that they can be stretched individually. Toe touches, for example, stretch both hamstrings; hurdlers' exercises stretch the hamstrings one at a time.

After endurance sports such as long-distance running, it is necessary to cool down by walking or jogging slowly. When we run for a long time in cross-country, for example, and then abruptly stop, blood pools in our legs, thereby decreasing the flow to our brains and causing light-headedness or fainting. We can prevent this by walking to cool down.

Athletes and Illness

EATING DISORDERS AND MENSTRUAL IRREGULARITY

Bulimia and anorexia nervosa are eating disorders. It is difficult to obtain exact figures for the incidence of these conditions, but some experts estimate that they may affect 10 percent of adolescent females. One study suggested that eating disorders affect one-third of female college athletes; another study suggested an incidence almost twice as great.

Anorexia is a disease manifested by avoidance of food, associated with an unnatural fear of gaining weight. Anorexic young women are painfully thin. They weigh less than 85 percent of their predicted body weight. The average female teen who is 5 feet tall should weigh 100 pounds; for each additional inch in height she should weigh 5 pounds more. An anorexic young woman at 5'6" tall would weigh less than 110 pounds rather than the expected 130 pounds. These girls can experience delayed onset or interruption of normal menstrual function.

Bulimia is binge eating followed by purging. This condition is more difficult to diagnose because the patients don't look overly thin. These patients will overeat at a meal and then excuse themselves from the table. They go to the bathroom and stick their fingers down their throats to induce vomiting. They may also take laxatives or fluid pills, fast, or exercise excessively to keep from gaining weight.

If the physician takes a thorough history, he or she can often diagnose an eating disorder. I ask the patient if she has lost weight during the last year and what she thinks her ideal weight should be. Patients with eating disorders will tell you an ideal weight that is significantly below the norms noted above. I ask about her menstrual history. If an athlete has not begun to menstruate by age sixteen or has begun to menstruate and then missed three consecutive periods or has three or fewer periods in a year, that causes me to suspect an eating disorder. Patients with eating disorders often complain of irregular bowel habits.

On a physical exam the most helpful indicators of an eating disorder are height and weight. Telltale signs of bulimia on a physical exam include an increased number of cavities (vomiting stomach acid destroys tooth enamel), an abnormal-looking fingernail on the index or middle finger of the dominant hand (stomach acid isn't good for nails, either), infections on the same fingers (for the same reason), and a chipmunk appearance of the cheeks (regurgitated acid inflames the salivary glands in the mouth).

Sports such as dance, running, and gymnastics emphasize thinness as an important ingredient of success. The emphasis on leanness encourages eating disorders and the resultant cessation of menses, which can lead to osteoporosis. If a teenage athlete has an eating disorder, she should see a physician. Other teens who are simply exercising excessively without the other hallmarks of an eating disorder and are not having periods should cut back on the intensity of their exercise. They will gain weight and menses should resume. If normal menstruation does not occur, these athletes should be treated with hormone replacement to prevent osteoporosis. Among teenaged girls with eating disorders, mental health consultation, hormonal therapy, calcium supplementation, and proper nutrition are all important interventions.

All teenage females should take calcium supplements whether or not they play sports. The recommended daily allowance of calcium for adolescent females is a 1000 milligrams per day. I tell my female teenage patients to take 500 milligrams of calcium supplement per day if they are menstruating and 1000 milligrams if they aren't having regular periods. Calcium supplements are available as either calcium carbonate or calcium citrate. Calcium carbonate is more commonly prescribed because it is less expensive, but calcium citrate is better absorbed. Increased absorption decreases the gastrointestinal complaints that sometimes accompany calcium supplementation. Patients often say to me that they don't want to take calcium supplements for fear of developing kidney stones. The fact is that although kidney stones contain calcium in most cases, taking calcium does not increase the risk of forming stones. One medical study found that people whose dietary calcium was increased actually formed fewer kidney stones than those taking less calcium.

Under most circumstances women strengthen their bones the most during their teenage years, and there is a continued increase in their bone density until they are thirty-five. At that time bone density begins to decrease gradually until menopause. After age thirty-five women lose approximately 1 percent of bone mass per year. The average age of menopause in the United States is fifty. After menopause bone loss occurs rapidly for approximately ten years. During this time women lose approximately 7 percent of their bone mass per year. Osteoporosis occurs in postmenopausal women because of this loss. In the athlete who is not having regular periods, bone density loss begins as a teen and can result in osteoporosis and stress fractures at a much younger age.

ANEMIA AND SICKLE-CELL DISEASE/TRAIT

What about *anemia* among athletes? It is common for athletes, particularly menstruating female teens, to be anemic as a result of iron deficiency. Some girls may complain of fatigue but others may have no symptoms at all. Anemia is caused by a decreased intake of dietary iron coupled with blood loss from menstrual flow. Anemia has a negative effect on performance in certain sports, especially those that require endurance.

The recommended daily allowance of iron for women is 15 milligrams per day, but the typical American diet supplies 5 milligrams of iron for each 1000 calories consumed. Therefore, a 100-pound cross-country runner would need to consume 3000 calories a day to achieve an adequate amount of iron intake. Even with the increased calorie expenditure from her training, she is not going to eat 3000 calories a day. The situation is complicated by the fact that the average woman loses approximately one ounce of blood each month from menstrual flow. Endurance runners lose additional blood from their intestinal tract as a result of training. Anemia is treated by oral iron supplements. (There is also a condition called *pseudoanemia* that occurs in endurance athletes. This abnormality is an increased volume of

ANEMIA HAS A NEGATIVE EFFECT ON PERFORMANCE IN CERTAIN SPORTS, ESPECIALLY THOSE THAT REQUIRE ENDURANCE.

fluid in the blood and can be found in routine blood testing. It is not really an illness and does not need to be treated.)

Making the correct diagnosis can be pretty complicated! Despite my general belief that laboratory tests are not particularly helpful when trying to screen asymptomatic athletes, I do test female teens for anemia because they are at increased risk for this condition. If your teenage daughter, especially one who competes in endurance sports, appears anemic, I recommend consulting a certified primary care sports medicine physician. These physicians can tell the difference between true anemia and pseudoanemia found in athletes.

Sickle-cell disease (or sickle-cell anemia) is an uncommon but serious condition that affects primarily African-Americans. It occurs in children who are homozygous for this condition. If you remember your Mendelian genetics from high school, you'll recall that if a person (or a green bean) has two different genes at a particular location, the individual is referred to as heterozygous for a trait. In this case only a dominant gene will express itself. If both genes are the same at a location, the condition is referred to as homozygous and the gene will express itself even if it is recessive rather than dominant. The sickle-cell gene is just such a recessive gene. Sickle-cell anemia is an abnormality of the red blood cells, which may sickle, or degenerate, clogging various organs so that they do not function. It can cause severe muscle pain, kidney failure, and even death.

A child with only one gene for sickle-cell disease is said to have *sickle-cell trait*. At one time this condition was considered to be harmless. Physicians thought that if there was only one gene for this condition, the problem wouldn't express itself and the red blood cells would be stable. In World War II African-American paratroopers with sickle-cell trait developed symptoms when they were flying at high altitudes similar to those of patients with sickle cell disease. We realized from this experience that sickle-cell trait could behave like true sickle-cell disease under certain conditions of physiological stress (so this condition does not truly behave like a Mendelian recessive trait).

In sports we see that youths with sickle-cell trait may develop symptoms of sickle-cell disease when they are dehydrated. As usual, prevention is the best treatment. African-American children should be tested for sickle-cell trait. If the test is positive, the parents should inform the coaches of this condition. Parents and coaches should take extra precautions so that these children don't get dehydrated (see the section on conditioning). These children should also avoid extreme exertion at high altitudes.

PERFORMANCE-ENHANCING DRUGS

The majority of athletes who use performance-enhancing drugs in college begin the drug use in high school, although fully one-third of these athletes begin using performance-enhancing drugs before high school. As many as 10 percent of male high school athletes use anabolic steroids to improve performance. These drugs work by building muscle, and they really work! Several years ago, before sports medicine researchers had adequately studied the effects of these agents, we erroneously told athletes that these drugs were only marginally effective in building muscle. This cost us a great deal of credibility with these athletes, because we now know that they are effective. They build strength and endurance, increase weight, speed recovery from muscle injury, and improve performance. They also have a large number of serious side effects: liver disease and jaundice, acne, breast development, violent mood changes, depression, tendon rupture, high blood pressure, elevated cholesterol, decreased sperm count, and atrophy of the testicles. They are also addictive. These drugs are banned by the National Football League, the International Olympic Committee, and the National Collegiate Athletic Association. Tell your children to stay away from them!

AS MANY AS 10 PERCENT OF MALE HIGH SCHOOL ATHLETES USE ANABOLIC STEROIDS TO IMPROVE PERFORMANCE.

A supplement widely used by young athletes is creatine. This substance is not banned and its sales have topped $100,000,000. Proponents of creatine say that it helps to build muscle, increase strength, and speed recovery from injury. But it can also cause dehydration, muscle cramps, and kidney trouble. I believe that physicians should discourage its use (and 85 percent of physician members of the Association of Professional Team Physicians also oppose its use) because we simply do not have enough information about its long-term safety or effectiveness.

Blood doping, which is withdrawing units of blood a few weeks before competition and then reinfusing them right before competition, is also illegal. Erythropoietin, which stimulates red blood cell production, and growth hormones are also used to enhance performance. Blood doping, erythropoietin, and growth hormones are not a problem among young athletes . . . yet.

DIET

Obesity is a major problem in our society. It is defined differently by different authorities, but most agree that when a child weighs 20 percent more than the recommended weight, he or she is overweight. Males should weigh 100 pounds if they are 5 feet tall and 6 pounds for every inch of height over 5 feet. A boy 5'10" should weigh 166 pounds. If he weighs 200 pounds, he has a weight problem. Thirty percent of adults are overweight. Eighty percent of overweight adolescents become overweight adults, but only 20 percent of overweight two-year-olds become obese adults. These numbers show that there is a window of opportunity to get overweight children to lose weight. We should try to normalize our children's weight between the time they are toddlers and the time they are teenagers. Although two-year-olds should not be put on a diet, we should make sure that toddlers are eating the right foods and in the right amounts. We should encourage our children to exercise regularly to keep their weight down. If they still have a weight problem by age ten, they can be placed on a carefully monitored diet. Kids, like adults, should get at least 55 percent of their calories from carbohydrates, no more than 30 percent from fat (of which only one-third, or 10 percent of the total, should be saturated fat), and the remaining 15 percent from protein.

Children should consume 15 calories per pound daily to maintain their weight. A 100-pound girl should consume 1500 calories to keep her weight at that level. Carbohydrates and protein contain 4 calories per gram. Fats contain 9 calories per gram. If we take in more calories than we burn, we gain weight, which is stored as fat. A pound of fat stores about 3500 calories. The above information forms the rudiments of any weight loss program.

Young athletes are inundated with advertisements and advice from friends about how to gain muscle or lose fat. There is a multimillion dollar industry built on food supplements and vitamins to help them accomplish this goal. Let's consider a couple of examples of how we can evaluate, on the basis of the above facts, the misinformation that your kids hear.

Your 120-pound fourteen-year-old son comes home from school and insists that you must immediately purchase creatine because his friend Johnny just gained 20 pounds of muscle using this product. What do you do? First, don't buy it. Johnny's interested in gaining weight and strength, so he began lifting weights. Second, Johnny's going through puberty. The male hormones, coupled with the weight training, are the reason for most of the gain in muscle mass. Johnny had to consume extra calories over and above what he needed for maintenance of his former weight in order to gain weight. These calories should come from eating more of the types of food that he normally eats.

Your sixteen-year-old daughter was injured skiing. She therefore missed the entire basketball season. The year before she was the starting point guard. She was 5'4" tall and weighed 120 pounds. When she was playing basketball, she consumed 2800 calories per day but didn't gain weight (120 pounds x 15 calories per pound = 1800 calories for maintenance, plus 1000 calories burned as a result of basketball practice and games). She has just gained 20 pounds in ten weeks because she continued to eat the same amount of food while burning far fewer calories as a result of inactivity from her injury. What does she do to lose the weight that she just gained?

Counting grams of fat is now in vogue, but I still prefer counting calories as long as the proportion of calories consumed from fats doesn't exceed 30 percent. Using the above data, we see that to maintain 120 pounds she needs to consume 1800 calories per day (120 pounds x 15 calories per pound) and to maintain 140 pounds she has been consuming 2100 calories per day (140 pounds x 15 calories per pound). We know that a pound of fat stores 3500 calories. Therefore, by eating between 1200 and 1500 calories per day she'll lose an additional pound per week because she will be eating about 500 calories less than maintenance per day for her weight (500 calories per day = 3500 calories per week = 1 pound of fat lost per week). Fortunately, your daughter's injury has healed and she has begun a jogging program that burns 500 calories per day. Using the same data we see that this translates to a weight loss of 1 additional pound per week. She can be back to 120 pounds in ten weeks with this combination of diet and exercise. Incidentally, if she eats 1500 calories per day and 30 percent of her calories comes from fat, she will be consuming 450 calories from fat. At 9 calories per gram this translates into 50 grams of fat per day. If this math is too complicated for you, consult with her physician or with Weight Watchers. The result should be the same.

Athletes also need to know *when* to eat. For the recreational athlete, eating after exercise makes sense. A phenomenon known as "afterburn" refers to the fact that after we exercise, our metabolism continues to run at an accelerated level, which allows us to burn calories faster than usual. Afterburn allows us to burn approximately 15 percent more calories when we eat after a walk rather than before one. I do not recommend *vigorous* exercise immediately after a meal. While we are digesting our food, blood is diverted from our muscles to our gastrointestinal tract to aid digestion. The blood supply won't be available to our muscles for vigorous exercise and to our intestine for digestion at the same time.

AFTER WE EXERCISE OUR METABOLISM CONTINUES TO RUN AT AN ACCELERATED LEVEL, WHICH ALLOWS US TO BURN CALORIES FASTER THAN USUAL.

Pregame meals for athletes should be eaten several hours before competition. The revered tradition of consuming fatty foods like steaks and eggs for a pregame meal is a bad idea. Carbohydrates are digested faster and more easily than fats, so they should make up the bulk of your child's pregame meal. Thus the ideal pregame meal is pasta or pancakes, not steak and eggs. Other carbohydrates that are ideal to consume before a game include rice, bread, and potatoes, but hold the sour cream.

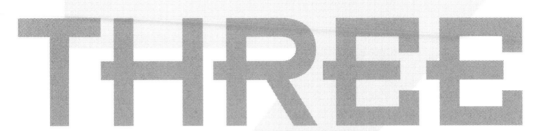

THREE

Treating

Athletic

Injuries

THE GENERAL TREATMENT OF ATHLETIC INJURIES

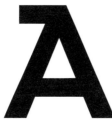thletic injuries are divided into two types, *acute injuries* and *overuse injuries*. An acute injury occurs all at once and is more likely to happen as a result of contact and collision or strenuous exercise. For example, a basketball player goes up for a rebound and comes down on another player's foot. She "rolls" her ankle. This is an ankle sprain, an acute injury. The vast majority of acute injuries that occur in youth sports are sprains, strains, and contusions. Patients often confuse the terminology, so let me give the medical definitions of these terms. A *sprain* is a ligament injury. A *ligament* is tissue that connects two bones. A *strain* is a muscle injury. A *contusion* is a bruise. These are usually not particularly serious injuries with long-term consequences. However, inadequate treatment of these problems may lead to a slower recovery and a lot of time lost from practice and games.

A SPRAIN IS A LIGAMENT INJURY. A LIGAMENT IS TISSUE THAT CONNECTS TWO BONES. A STRAIN IS A MUSCLE INJURY. A CONTUSION IS A BRUISE.

Overuse injuries, on the other hand, are rarely due to contact. They are more likely to result from recurrent minor trauma. For example, a football player begins a jogging program in order to get in shape by the time practice starts in six weeks. He has been a couch potato since basketball season ended, so he runs five miles a day every day to get in shape faster. One month after he begins this program he has pain in the lower leg. He is developing medial tibial stress syndrome, an overuse injury. It is a process, not an event. Typically the pain first comes on after a run. If the athlete ignores the pain and continues to train, the pain will come on during a run. Finally, if the athlete persists in training, the pain will occur at rest.

It has been estimated that half of all youth sports injuries result from overuse rather than from acute trauma. Most of these injuries involve the lower extremities. Some also occur in the dominant arms of athletes involved in sports that require throwing.

There are many factors that lead to overuse injuries. Training errors are a major contributing factor. When our children abruptly increase either the intensity or duration of their workouts, they injure themselves. I recommend an increase of approximately 10 percent effort every couple of weeks to avoid overtraining. Take, for example, a cross-country runner. She wants to increase her distance and is training with five-mile runs three days a week along with her long-distance and interval training. I tell her to increase the distance to five and one-half miles and keep the same pace for two weeks before making another incremental increase.

TREATMENT OF OVERUSE INJURIES DEPENDS ON HOW FAR THE INJURY HAS PROGRESSED AT THE TIME OF DIAGNOSIS.

Treatment of overuse injuries depends on how far the injury has progressed at the time of diagnosis. If we catch these problems early, they are easier to treat. If the football player mentioned above is diagnosed when he has pain after his training run, I prescribe ice, stretching, and a 20 percent reduction in training. For example, I tell him to decrease the training run from five to four miles per day. If I don't see the athlete until he has pain while he is running, I advise ice, stretching, and a 50 percent reduction in the training program. If an athlete doesn't come to me until he is having pain at rest, I prescribe a week off from training and the administration of non-steroidal anti-inflammatory agents, as well as ice and stretching. If an athlete has to avoid training for one week or longer as a result of an overuse injury, I advise cross-training to maintain cardiovascular fitness. For example, if a high school runner can't run, I tell her to ride the stationary bike, swim, or run in the swimming pool in chest-deep water until she can return to training for her event. I encourage her to do these alternative exercises at the same level of intensity that she would normally use for running, and for the same duration.

The most common injury is reinjury. Once your child has an injury, be certain that the problem is thoroughly corrected before you allow him to return to his sport. Before the child returns to competition, the injured joint should be as mobile as its noninjured counterpart and 80 to 90 percent as strong.

As noted in the chapter on conditioning, most injuries occur during the fall sports season because kids are out of shape when they come to camp for their fall sport. Parents and coaches, be careful! Go slowly at first!

! Tips for coaches:

Give your athletes a training program for the summer. Test them when they return in the fall to ensure that they are ready for the next level of training. This will prevent not only overuse injuries but heat injuries as well.

Parents and coaches can initiate treatment for athletic injuries immediately after they occur by utilizing the R.I.C.E. protocol—*rest, ice, compression, and elevation.* This treatment promotes more rapid healing and gets the athlete back to competition more quickly. When tissue is injured, fluid leaks from the blood vessels, causing swelling. This process begins immediately after the injury occurs and can continue for up to seventy-two hours. We can minimize the effect of swelling by using R.I.C.E.

! Tips for coaches:

If you don't take anything else away from this book, learn the following and you can successfully treat 90 percent of the injuries that you encounter.

- REST the injured part. A child who sprains his or her ankle should get off it. Physicians currently advocate not complete rest but *relative rest.* In the case of a severe sprain we may have to put a patient on crutches for a couple of days, but we do this for a shorter time than we did a few years ago. Healing occurs faster if the athlete bears weight on the injured limb as soon as possible. Injured players should avoid activities that cause pain but should still perform other exercises, including those that promote cardio-vascular fitness, such as rowing, cycling, or swimming. They also should work on flexibility by performing stretching exercises. The athletes can return to competition when they have a pain-free range of motion (i.e., flexibility) of the affected area that is equal to the range of the uninjured side and when the injured area is 80 to 90 percent as strong as the unaffected side.
- ICE the affected area. This limits the leakage of fluid from the capillaries, which are small blood vessels. Use an ice pack with crushed ice that molds itself to the area to which it is applied. If it's more convenient, simply grab a bag of frozen vegetables from

the freezer and apply it to the injured area. Either of these will mold itself to the injured site. I also fill a bunch of Styrofoam cups with water and put them in the freezer. I tell athletes with injuries to peel about one inch of the Styrofoam from the top of the cup and rub the affected area with the ice. This allows them to hold the insulated cup while applying ice to the injury. Apply ice for twenty minutes as often as you think about it. Use ice as often as every two hours but at least three times a day for the first forty-eight hours. Place a towel between the skin and the ice pack to protect the skin against cold injury. Heat may make an acute injury feel better, but never use it until all signs of inflammation go away! I advise withholding heat for at least the first three to five days after an acute injury.

- COMPRESS the injured area with an elastic bandage or splint to further limit swelling. Be sure not to wrap the injured area too tightly.
- ELEVATE the injured part above the level of the heart to promote the drainage of fluids away from the injury, utilizing gravity.

I also advise the use of an analgesic (pain reliever), such as acetaminophen (Tylenol), or an analgesic/anti-inflammatory agent (reduces injury), such as ibuprofen (Advil), for pain and inflammation. The latter drugs are analgesic at low doses (e.g., two tablets three times a day) and don't have an anti-inflammatory effect unless used at higher doses. The anti-inflammatory dose of ibuprofen in an adult is 2400 milligrams, or twelve tablets per day. For children, the anti-inflammatory dose depends on the child's weight. Consult your physician before using anti-inflammatory doses of this or other medications. Many sports medicine experts are reluctant to use ibuprofen and other anti-inflammatory drugs in children and adolescents because of concern over Reye's syndrome, an often fatal disease that has been observed in some children after they have taken aspirin. However, it has not been associated with other anti-inflammatory drugs, and I do not hesitate to prescribe these drugs when there is a medical indication for their use.

After the inflammation has gone away, it's time to employ another R, rehabilitation. When we rehabilitate an injured area, we first concentrate on flexibility, and then on strength. One regains flexibility of the injured area by performing range-of-motion exercises. One of the things that makes the diagnosis in sports injuries easier is that most of the structures in our body are mirror images of another structure on the opposite side. For example, when I see a child with an injured left knee, I always examine the right knee first. This gives me a reasonably good idea of what is normal for that individual. Regaining full flexibility means that the injured left knee can move as well as the uninjured right knee. Comparing the injured and uninjured sides also aids in determining how strong the injured side is. The injured athlete can improve strength by performing resistance exercises such as weight lifting. The athlete should not return to practice until the injured side is as flexible as the uninjured side and 80 to 90 percent as strong as the uninjured side.

Despite advances in equipment, rules, and technique, injury is part of sport, especially contact and collision sports. The best safeguards against injury are to have the athletes well conditioned and warmed up before competition, to make sure that the coaches and players know the rules and that they are enforced, and to make sure that the equipment fits properly. At the novice levels of competition, where coaches, managers, and officials are less experienced, parents often have to oversee these safety issues.

A physician should be in attendance at all athletic contests that involve contact or collision on the junior high level and higher. This is easier to achieve than you might think because certified sports medicine physicians are all sports junkies anyway and are looking for an excuse to attend one more sporting event. If this fails, contact a parent in your school who is a physician. If this doesn't work, call the local teaching hospital with a family practice residency or sports medicine fellowship, and ask if one of the residents in training will serve as team physician.

Head and Neck Injuries

HEAD INJURIES

Serious head injuries occur almost exclusively as a result of playing contact and collision sports such as football and ice hockey. Boxing can cause many head injuries, but this does not occur often at the youth level because the aim of Olympic and Golden Gloves boxing is to outpoint rather than disable your opponent. Among the remaining contact and collision sports, football is responsible for the vast majority of serious head injuries because of the large number of participants and because the helmeted head is often used as the initial point of contact.

A *concussion* is a potentially serious head injury suffered in contact sports. This is a common injury affecting approximately a quarter of a million athletes per year. A concussion is defined as a temporary alteration in brain function without an associated anatomical change. In football parlance it's anything from "getting your bell rung" to getting "knocked out." A player shaken up after a hit will come out of the game under his own power but can't tell you what quarter is being played or what the last play was. A player who has recently come out of the game may be simply sitting on the bench staring out into space or he may complain that he just doesn't feel right. He may also complain of headaches or blurry vision. To check the mental status of a player on the sideline the physician will ask him to perform serial sevens or three-object recall. Serial sevens involves counting backward from one hundred by sevens (93, 86, 79, 72, etc.). Three-object recall involves naming three objects (e.g., stop sign, tennis ball, and screen door) and then asking the athlete to tell you what these objects were after five minutes has passed.

There are several ways to classify a concussion. The Colorado Medical Society suggests a very practical way of grading concussions that facilitates making a decision about whether the affected athlete should return to play. Its guidelines have become a national standard for treating players who have suffered a concussion. Most team physicians use these or other similar guidelines. All athletes who suffer their first concussion should be immediately removed from play and evaluated on the sidelines by a physician.

- A *grade I concussion* involves confusion but no loss of consciousness and no amnesia. Once the confusion has cleared, the player may return to participation if he or she is asymptomatic for twenty minutes.
- A *grade II concussion* involves confusion with amnesia but no loss of consciousness. A player with a grade II concussion may return to practice or competition after being asymptomatic for one week.
- A *grade III concussion* involves a loss of consciousness. Players who sustain a grade III concussion may return to competition after one month, as long as they have no symptoms (e.g., headache) for two weeks before competing.

After a second concussion of any grade, the athlete must be withheld from play for a longer time. Recurrent concussions can be season- or even career-ending injuries. A player who has had a concussion is four times as likely to have a second concussion as an athlete who has never sustained one.

Learn the ABCs for treating an unconscious person. Whenever you come upon an unconscious athlete, if you're the first to arrive, check the following:

- *Airway:* Check to make sure that the player hasn't swallowed grass or a mouthpiece that could obstruct his or her breathing.
- *Breathing:* Make sure that the person is breathing.
- *Circulation:* Check the pulse to make certain that the heart is pumping blood effectively.

After you have checked the ABCs, take these steps:

- If the patient is not breathing or circulating blood, begin CPR, if you know how.
- If the ABCs are all OK, don't move the patient; kneel and hold the neck stationary until the rescue squad comes.
- In all cases of a head- or neck-injured player, make sure that someone has called 911.

A very dangerous situation that can occur after head trauma is called *second impact syndrome*. This happens when an athlete sustains a head injury and returns to competition too soon. He can sustain a second minor head trauma and become unconscious because the first injury has caused brain swelling and the athlete returns to play before the swelling has gone down. The second trauma can then prove fatal. The lesson here is clear. *Withhold your child from games and practice after a head injury, no matter how trivial it seems, and seek medical attention from a sports medicine physician.* We can prevent catastrophic head injuries by treating the less severe ones appropriately.

WITHHOLD YOUR CHILD FROM GAMES AND PRACTICE AFTER A HEAD INJURY, NO MATTER HOW TRIVIAL IT SEEMS, AND SEEK MEDICAL ATTENTION FROM A SPORTS MEDICINE PHYSICIAN.

One of the major causes of head injuries is the failure to wear helmets while biking. Though not many of our children cycle competitively, they often ride bikes for recreation. Be prepared for the inevitable fall and insist that your children wear helmets. Don't just encourage them. Show them by your example.

Serious head injuries in contact sports such as boxing and football can also be lessened by wearing mouth guards. They absorb some of the shock when a contestant is hit on the chin. Therefore, the full effect of the blow is not transmitted to the brain. Parents, insist that your children wear a mouthpiece at all times. They protect their brains as well as their teeth. I suggest a mouthpiece for all contact and collision sports, including basketball.

NECK INJURIES

The protective equipment worn by football players is a double-edged sword as far as neck injuries are concerned. Helmets and shoulder pads lessen some types of injuries but make other injuries more likely. The helmet protects the head from trauma but also encourages players to use their helmeted heads as weapons, thereby increasing the likelihood of serious neck injuries. Such injuries have become less likely in the wake of rule changes outlawing spearing—the use of a helmet rather than a shoulder as the primary point of contact in tackling. Spearing was responsible for severe paralyzing injuries to the player making the tackle.

Many neck injuries occur to players who have a narrower-than-normal spinal canal, making a spinal cord damaging injury more likely. It is not practical for all youth players, or even all professional players, to be screened for this condition by performing an MRI (magnetic resonance imaging) scan. If a player does sustain an injury in which there is temporary loss of neuromuscular function, he or she should have an MRI scan to check for a narrow spinal canal. If the scan demonstrates an abnormally small spinal canal, the athlete should quit playing contact and collision sports. If the youth continues to play, he or she is at risk for a paralyzing injury because compression of the spinal cord is more likely if the spinal canal is narrow.

As with head injuries, we can do some things to prevent serious neck injuries as well. Players in the weight room should be encouraged to work on neck-strengthening exercises. Players are too concerned about how much they can bench or squat, but they should concentrate more on their neck muscles in order to avoid serious injury. Coaches should devote sufficient time to instructing their players in proper tackling and blocking techniques, making sure that players do not tackle with their helmets.

A *burner* or *stinger* is a common, less severe neck injury that is often confused with the more severe paralyzing injuries mentioned above. In one study of college football players, two-thirds of the participants reported having a burner during their playing career.

A player suffers a burner either when he is struck directly on the shoulder, lowering it and stretching the nerves from the neck to the shoulder and arm in an area that we call the brachial plexus, or when the nerve is pinched as a result of a direct hit on the top of the head. It is easy to tell when an athlete sustains his first burner. He runs off the field holding his arm limp as if he had just been shot. The player experiences numbness and tingling that shoots down the affected arm, and in severe cases, he will have weakness as well. The player should be withheld from competition while symptoms last but may return to the game as soon as strength and sensation return to normal. Some players suffer from repeated burners and may have to be fitted with special equipment to prevent recurrences. These players are given a collar or special pads called shock pads that are worn underneath their regular shoulder pads. A player who suffers repeated burners should also do extra neck- and shoulder-strengthening exercises to prevent recurrences. Burners are sometimes a result of improper blocking or tackling technique that must be corrected. They are usually limited to one side or the other. If a player complains of weakness or numbness and tingling in both arms, suspect a more serious neck injury. Don't let the athlete return to competition and promptly seek medical attention.

SUMMARY

Head and neck injuries are the most serious ones in contact sports. Whenever I stand on the sidelines at a high school football game and see a player go down with a head or neck injury, I cringe. I'm certain that at youth games, where there is rarely a physician around, the parents wince even more. Here are some guidelines for parents and coaches to follow when faced with the sudden necessity to deal with these injuries:

- Most important, don't move the injured player who either is unconscious or has sustained a neck injury. I have watched professional football games on national television in which unconscious players were removed from the field of play without having their necks stabilized. It is often moving a player with an unstable spinal injury, rather than the initial trauma, that is responsible for subsequent paralysis.
- Don't move any player who is complaining of severe neck pain, tingling, or numbness in the arms or legs.
- Always know where the nearest phone is to call 911!

- Never be embarrassed about stopping play while waiting for competent medical personnel to arrive to attend to the injuries of a player suspected of having a severe head or neck injury. It is always better to halt play until an ambulance arrives and emergency personnel can carefully and appropriately remove an injured player than to risk further injury by moving him or her.

Facial Injuries

EYE INJURIES

Injuries to the eyes are uncommon in baseball, football, and lacrosse and are becoming less frequent in ice hockey because of the protection afforded by helmets. Visors incorporated into the face masks of the helmets further reduce the incidence of eye injuries and permit an injured player to compete without risking further injury. These injuries were very common in the past, and their frequency led to the development of state-of-the-art helmets. The letters NOCSAE in any football helmet indicate that it has been manufactured according to exacting safety standards. Football and lacrosse helmets have four-point fixation, which means that the helmet has two straps on each side so that it won't slip up and down. Ice hockey helmets, on the other hand, have only one strap on each side and are more likely to slip. When this happens, the front of the helmet strikes the nose, often causing an injury such as nasal laceration.

Sport goggles containing polycarbonate lenses or contact lenses should be worn by any contestants in contact and collision sports who would otherwise wear glasses while participating. I advise against wearing extended wear contact lenses because they pose an increased risk of corneal infection.

The commonest eye injury is a corneal abrasion that occurs when a participant is struck in the eye by an opponent's finger. This type of injury is more common in sports such as basketball, soccer, or rugby, contact sports in which players don't wear protective equipment. The injured athlete complains of a gritty or sandy feeling in the eye. The diagnosis is made by the physician, who applies fluorescein dye to the eye to demonstrate the abrasion. Treatment consists of resting and sometimes patching the eye for a short period of time, usually twenty-four hours. Participants playing racquet sports in close quarters (e.g., squash and racquetball) should wear protective goggles to prevent eye trauma.

Another less common but more severe injury is a *blow-out fracture of the orbit.* This is a fracture of the very thin bone that makes up the floor of the eye socket. This type of injury occurs when a player is struck in the eye with a ball. The eyeball is compressed, and the force is transmitted to this bone, fracturing it. The diagnosis of a blow-out fracture of the orbit is suggested when the player complains of double vision after eye trauma. The physician may have the player follow a moving finger with her eyes while she holds her head still. If the eyes don't track in unison, then a blow-out fracture is likely. The diagnosis is made by taking an x-ray of the facial bones. Treatment is surgical correction by an ophthalmologist or plastic surgeon.

Another eye condition is *chemical conjunctivitis,* often suffered by swimmers as a result of irritation from the chlorine in the water. The symptoms are redness and stinging of the eyes. A prescription medicine called Acular, in eyedrop form, is used to treat this problem. Swimmers can also get *bacterial conjunctivitis,* whose symptoms are a thick milky discharge from the eye and the redness and burning similar to chemical conjunctivitis. It is important to distinguish between these two conditions because bacterial conjunctivitis, which is treated with topical antibiotics, is very contagious. Swimmers must stay out of the pool while they have it.

EAR INJURIES

Ear injuries occur most often in wrestling and boxing. The so-called *cauliflower ear* occurs as a result of shearing forces across the ear that cause bleeding and the formation of blood clots between the skin and the cartilage. When this injury occurs, seek prompt medical attention. If the blood is not drained, disfiguring scarring can occur. As with most injuries, the best treatment is prevention. Properly fitting headgear will protect boxers and wrestlers from this type of injury.

Swimmer's ear is a condition that affects only a small group of athletes. It may sound like a trivial problem but can be so painful as to be disabling. I advise swimmers to mix equal quantities of rubbing alcohol and vinegar and put a couple of drops in each ear after practice and competition to prevent this bacterial infection. Certain well-fitting earplugs or Silly Putty is protective. Prescription eardrops are used to treat the infection. A child with swimmer's ear can hasten recovery by using a hair dryer to dry the ear canals upon emerging from the water after swim practice.

Many children have had pressure-equalizing tubes surgically implanted in their ears. I'm often asked if these devices present a problem during swimming and diving. I see no problem swimming with the tubes in place, but diving can be a problem. Again, custom-fitted earplugs or a wad of Silly Putty molded to fit the contour of the ear canal can be helpful in divers with pressure-equalizing tubes in place.

NASAL INJURIES

A bloody nose is a very common but not particularly severe injury. It can be correctly diagnosed and usually treated by a parent on the sideline of the athletic contest. In this era of concern over blood-borne infections, the player with a nosebleed or any other source of bleeding should be immediately removed from competition. Pinch the nose to compress the ruptured blood vessel and apply ice to constrict the bleeding blood vessel. Many people recommend having the injured player tilt the head backwards, but this causes blood to run down the back of the throat, causing nausea. I advise players to hold their heads in a neutral position and spit out the blood rather than swallow it. It is necessary, of course, to observe universal blood and body fluid precautions while doing this. This means that all blood and blood-soaked clothing must be kept from contacting another player or spectator. Bleeding usually stops in about fifteen minutes. If the bleeding doesn't stop, consult a physician, who will pack the nose and sometimes apply medications to cause the blood vessels to constrict. The packing can be removed in a couple of days. Nasal fractures are common in sports. They are almost never a serious problem. Apply ice for twenty minutes every hour or two and consult an ear, nose, and throat surgeon, who will usually wait about forty-eight hours to allow the swelling to decrease before reducing the fracture. The cosmetic and functional results are excellent.

Five percent of the visits that young athletes make to physicians' offices are for sinus infections. These are particularly frequent among swimmers and can be treated with antibiotics.

ORAL AND DENTAL INJURIES

I urge soccer and basketball players to wear mouthpieces while competing. Not only does this protect them, but it also diminishes the chances of transmitting a bloodborne infection in the event they are struck in the mouth by another player's elbow or fist. I am not an expert on dentistry, but as a sports medicine and team physician I have seen my share of dental injuries. If your child loses a tooth as a result of a sports injury, soak the tooth in milk to remove debris. Don't scrub the tooth. Contact your dentist immediately. If you cannot see a dentist within a half hour, try to reimplant the tooth in its socket yourself. Teeth that are reimplanted within thirty minutes are more likely to be successfully revived than those done later. Face masks and mouth guards have reduced the incidence of dental injuries substantially.

Arm Injuries

SHOULDER INJURIES

There are two common shoulder injuries that occur as a result of a collision. The first is a *shoulder dislocation;* the second is *shoulder separation.* The shoulder is one of the easiest joints in the body to dislocate. The head of the humerus (the long bone of the upper arm) is relatively large and sits in the relatively shallow socket of the shoulder (the hip, by contrast, has a deeper socket) (Fig. 1). Because of this relationship, only about one-third of the humoral head is in contact with the shoulder socket at any time. Therefore, a blow to the arm can dislodge the bone from its socket, causing a dislocation.

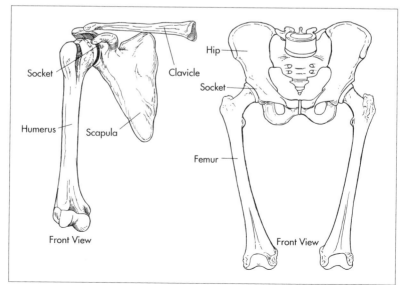

FIGURE 1 SHOULDER AND HIP SOCKETS

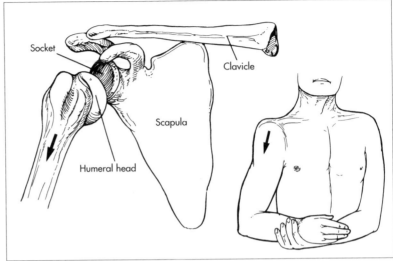

FIGURE 2 ANTERIOR SHOULDER DISLOCATION

There are two common types of shoulder dislocations: the *anterior* dislocation and the *posterior* dislocation. Ninety-five percent of shoulder dislocations are anterior dislocations (Fig. 2). This injury typically occurs in a contact sport when a defensive player attempts to arm tackle a ball carrier, or a falling player breaks his or her fall by extending an arm out to the side. The impact pushes the arm back and the ball-shaped head of the humerus pops forward out of the socket. With this type of injury it is relatively easy to put the shoulder back in place. Physicians use several different methods to reduce or relocate the anterior dislocated shoulder. The method I prefer is to bring the patient to the emergency department and obtain x-rays to make certain that there are no other associated injuries. Next, I give the patient some intravenous sedation and have him or her lie face down on a stretcher. I then apply a weight around the patient's wrist. The force of the weight in the sedated patient whose muscles are relaxed usually provides enough force to reduce the dislocation. After an anterior dislocation, a player can return to play in a few weeks if he is fitted with a protective brace that limits motion of the arm at the shoulder. This will prevent further dislocations. Some players suffer repeated anterior shoulder dislocations and require surgery to tighten the muscles, which have become lax as a result of these repeated injuries. Posterior dislocations are much less common and are rarely seen in youth sports. In a posterior dislocation the arm bone is forcibly driven out of the back side of the joint.

A shoulder separation is another, much less serious injury, which occurs when a player falls or is struck directly on the shoulder. Shoulder pads, which do nothing to prevent dislocations, do protect against separations. When this injury occurs, the ligaments between the acromion (the upper portion of the scapula, or shoulder blade) and the collarbone are stretched and sometimes torn. A shoulder separation is really a sprain.

The following classification of shoulder sprains applies to all ligamentous sprains. Shoulder separations, or sprains, are divided into first-degree (mild) sprains, in which there is stretching of the fibers of the ligament without a tear; second-degree (moderate) sprains, in which the fibers are partially torn; and third-degree (severe) sprains, in which the ligament is completely torn (Fig. 3).

Mild and moderate separations do not require surgical correction. Even most third-degree sprains can be treated conservatively without resorting to surgery. The major benefit of surgery in a third-degree sprain is to correct the appearance of the shoulder. Team physicians will often allow players to compete with a first-degree separation if there is not too much discomfort and the injury is properly padded. The important consideration is the

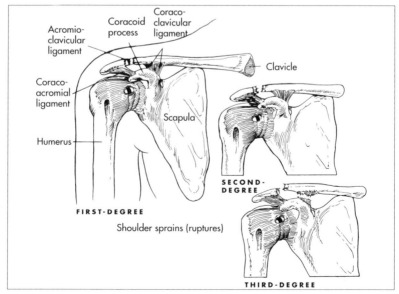

FIGURE 3 FIRST-DEGREE, SECOND-DEGREE, AND THIRD-DEGREE SHOULDER SPRAINS

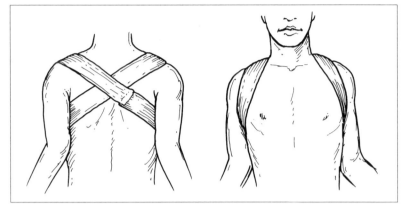

FIGURE 4 FIGURE-OF-EIGHT STRAP

player's comfort. There is very little risk of the injury's becoming more severe if the athlete with minimal symptoms continues to compete. We must apply some common sense and consider the situation. I would not allow a twelve-year-old lacrosse player to participate in a game with a first-degree shoulder separation, but I would allow a senior in high school to participate in the city championship with the same injury.

The only common fracture in the shoulder region that we see in sports is the *fractured collarbone,* or *clavicle.* These fractures usually result from a fall directly on the shoulder. It is most commonly the midportion of the bone that is broken. These injuries usually heal very well if the physician applies a figure-of-eight strap around the athlete's shoulders for three to six weeks (Fig. 4).

It should be worn continuously while the fracture heals. There is often a significant lump in the midshaft of the clavicle after the fracture heals. As time passes, the bone remodels and the lump disappears. This is particularly true the younger the athlete is at the time of the injury. There are other, more severe fractures involving the shoulder and upper arm, but these are extremely rare in sports other than motor sports.

There are other shoulder injuries that result from repeated microtrauma rather than from one traumatic event. These injuries are called *overuse injuries.* One such injury is *Little League shoulder,* which results from repeated microtrauma from throwing that leads to a stress fracture at the growth plate (Fig. 5). Children also suffer from instability of the shoulder musculature. Your child may complain of a feeling of looseness or instability of the arm while throwing, or he or she may say that the arm feels

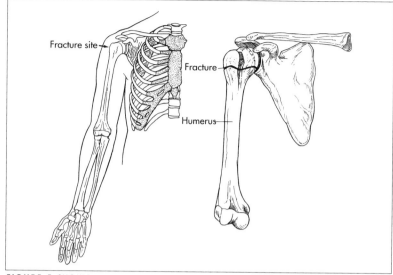

FIGURE 5 SHOULDER STRESS FRACTURE: LITTLE LEAGUE SHOULDER

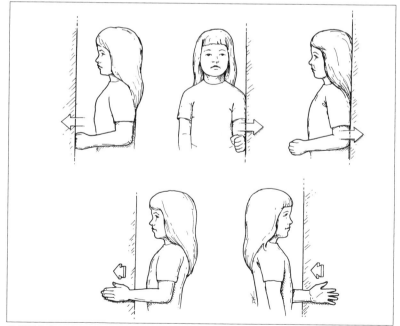

FIGURE 6 MUSCLE-STRENGTHENING EXERCISES

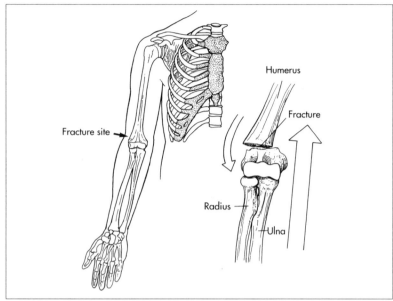

FIGURE 7 ELBOW FRACTURE DISLOCATION

"dead." The apprehension test can establish the diagnosis. In this test, pressure is placed on the shoulder from behind, causing apprehension in the athlete that the shoulder will pop out of place. The shoulder is then pushed backwards from the front of the joint, and the athlete feels a sense of relief. This injury is treated with relative rest, which in this case means restraining of throwing. Muscle-strengthening exercises such as isometrically pushing against a door jam help strengthen the shoulder musculature and are a useful treatment (Fig. 6).

ELBOW INJURIES

Acute injuries around the elbow are rare in youth sports. In my twenty-one years of family medical practice with a special interest in sports medicine, I have seen more elbow dislocations as a result of children falling out of trees than in all sports combined. However, an elbow *fracture dislocation* can be a true medical emergency. This injury involves both a fracture (broken bone) and a dislocation (displaced fragment). It typically occurs when a player falls with the elbow locked (Fig. 7). The injury is serious because it can damage the nerve and artery that cross the joint. I always feel the pulse and assess the color and temperature of the hand to ensure that there is no damage to the blood supply. If the hand is cold, blue, and pulseless, call 911 because this is a *limb-threatening* injury! Do not attempt to reduce the dislocation yourself because you may cause further damage.

Another traumatic elbow injury is the *hyperextended elbow,* which occurs when a player attempts to tackle another player. The tackler is injured as he involuntarily straightens his forearm. The patient will complain of pain when he or she straightens the elbow or bends the elbow against resistance. The usual recovery time is a few days for mild injuries and up to three or four weeks for more severe injuries. In less severe injuries no treatment is necessary. In the more severe hyperextension elbow injuries, treatment consists of resting the arm in a sling for a few days until the severe pain is gone. The athlete then begins range-of-motion exercises to increase the pain-free motion of the elbow. Finally, he or she will exercise against resistance—for example, by lifting weights—to build strength.

Two other elbow injuries are the *tennis elbow* and the *Little League elbow.* Both are overuse injuries that occur after repeated microtrauma rather than after an acute injury. The typical tennis elbow injury occurs as a result of snapping the wrist while hitting the backhand shot. The proper technique involves hitting with the wrist rigid in a neutral position. If a player extends the wrist while hitting, there is an inordinate pull on the tendon that attaches on the outside of the elbow joint. Inflammation of the tendon occurs when a player does this repeatedly. Hitting off center or with an oversized racket or one that is too tightly strung also contributes to this type of injury. Treatment is to ice the outside of the elbow before and after playing and to take ibuprofen or a similar medication. A tennis elbow strap, which can be purchased at an ortho-

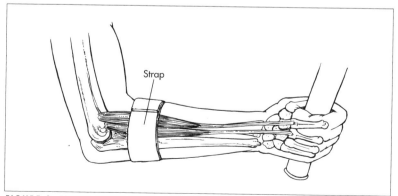

Strap

FIGURE 8 TENNIS ELBOW STRAP

pedic supply store or sports store, is also helpful. This strap is worn on the forearm, below the elbow, not on the elbow itself (Fig. 8). It prevents complete tightening of the muscle that attaches on the outside of the elbow. I advise players to wear the strap each time they play tennis until the symptoms subside. Change to a racket with a smaller head or a less tightly strung racket if equipment is the problem. Stretching and strengthening exercises can be done to relieve symptoms (Fig. 9). If this treatment fails, the player will have to take some time off from tennis or at least avoid hitting the backhand shot until symptoms disappear. If the pain persists, a physician can inject the area with cortisone compound. A player must avoid playing for one week after the injection. Surgery is rarely necessary. Elite tennis players develop a tennis elbow on the inside of the elbow rather than the outside. This results from snapping the wrist inward to impart spin while serving.

Little League elbow occurs only among youth players. On the inside of a young player's elbow there is a soft area of cartilage within the bone that is the site of bone growth. This structure is subject to stress when the ball is thrown. A single pitch never causes this type of injury. If a young player throws too many pitches, he or she can sustain a fracture of the growth plate and actually tear off a piece of bone (Fig. 10).

The treatment for this injury is rest for six to twelve weeks before the pitcher can return to play. This usually means that the player is lost for the season. Since this growth center is closed by

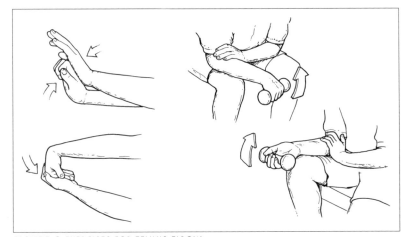

FIGURE 9 EXERCISES FOR TENNIS ELBOW

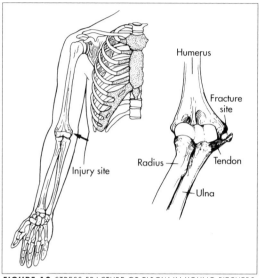

FIGURE 10 STRESS FRACTURE OF ELBOW IN YOUNG PITCHERS

Humerus

Fracture site

Tendon

Radius

Ulna

Injury site

age fifteen, we don't see this injury in older players. Little League, in its wisdom, limits to six the number of innings that a pitcher can pitch in one week, a policy that reduces the frequency of this injury. The Little League rules state that, "if a player pitches in four or more innings, three calendar days of rest must be observed."

These rules help, but parents still need to be vigilant to make sure that their children are not throwing too many pitches. For example, I would recommend monitoring the total number of pitches thrown. If a pitcher is struggling, he or she might throw 30 pitches per inning. In a six-inning game, this would add up to 180 pitches! It is difficult to say exactly how many pitches a young pitcher should throw in a particular game. There are many variables to consider, such as how many days the pitcher has rested since his or her last outing and whether the weather is hot or cold. It is less damaging to the arm to pitch in hot weather than it is to pitch in cold weather. The pitcher also has to be particularly careful at the beginning of the season after a long winter layoff. As a general recommendation I would limit a Little League pitcher to 50 or 60 pitches early in the season; that number could increase gradually to 70 or 80 toward the season's end. High school pitchers should also start out gradually and then increase the pitch count. In most situations I wouldn't let a pitcher throw more than 100 pitches in an outing. This is particularly true north of the Mason-Dixon line, where the season begins when the weather is still quite cold.

FOREARM INJURIES

The only common injury of the forearm is the so-called *billy club* or *nightstick fracture* of the midportion of the forearm. This injury got its name because it most often occurred when a person raised his or her hand to protect the face from a blow from a police officer's nightstick. In sports it most frequently occurs in football when a player is struck in the forearm by an opponent's helmet. These injuries almost always heal without surgery but require eight to ten weeks of immobilization in a cast rather than the six weeks that is the standard for many other fractures. Parents, if your child comes out of a football game complaining of pain in the middle of the forearm on the side of the little finger (not the thumb side), assume that he has a fracture. If the pain persists, get him to a physician for an x-ray, but don't get talked into surgery until you talk to a sports medicine expert.

WRIST INJURIES

Wrist injuries are very common in younger athletes. They can occur in both contact and noncontact sports, when the child falls on the outstretched hand. Fractures that occur in the wrist usually involve the end of one or both of the long bones of the forearm rather than the wrist bones themselves. A child who falls on the outstretched arm will complain of pain and will often have an obvious bump on the back of the wrist. Wrist fractures are reduced and immobilized in a cast, which goes from the fingers to above the elbow, for four to six weeks. They heal nicely. Older children sustain a *Colles fracture*, in which the bone is actually broken (Fig. 11). Younger children sustain a *buckle fracture*, in which the bone is partially collapsed (like a soda can that has been stepped on). This fracture is less serious and heals in a shorter time.

Occasionally, one of the wrist bones, called the *scaphoid navicular,* fractures in the same kind of fall. This injury is initially difficult to diagnose and is often missed on

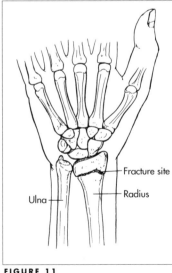

Ulna

Fracture site

Radius

FIGURE 11
COLLES FRACTURE OF THE WRIST

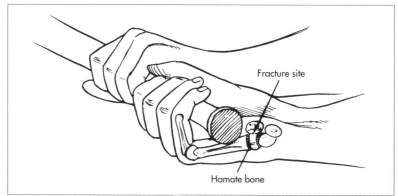

FIGURE 12 HAMATE (FRACTURED BY REPEATED BATTING)

the initial x-ray. If your child has severe or persistent wrist pain after a fall, consult with a sports medicine specialist. The doctor will repeat the x-ray after about a week. By this time, a fracture line is evident on the x-ray, and the diagnosis is easily made. The fracture often requires 12 weeks to heal. It requires casting, which immobilizes the thumb as well as the wrist and elbow joint.

As children age, their bones become stronger. A seven-year-old soccer player may fracture his or her wrist in a fall, whereas the sixteen-year-old tennis player may only sprain his or her wrist in the same kind of fall. The wrist sprain takes two to three weeks to heal. The most common overuse injury to the wrist occurs among the largest and the most petite athletes that I see in my practice. Gymnasts experience wrist overuse injuries because they bear their entire body weight on their extended wrists. Football offensive linemen also suffer these injuries because they are pushing two-hundred-pound defensive linemen with their arms extended. In either case, if these athletes have wrist pain, they have to modify their training regimen to avoid the activity that causes the pain until symptoms resolve. This often takes several weeks.

A young baseball player can fracture a wrist bone called the *hamate*. This bone has a hook on it that sticks up in the palm of the hand. As a result of repeatedly hitting a ball with the bat, the player can fracture this hook (Fig. 12). If your child has pain on the palm side of the hand near the skin crease of the wrist, suspect this injury.

Carpal tunnel syndrome is a common overuse injury that affects the wrists. It occurs when the median nerve going down the arm to the hand is trapped as it traverses the wrist. This is a particularly common injury in wheelchair-bound athletes because of the enormous stress placed on the wrists to propel the wheelchair. Patients complain of pain or numbness and tingling in the first three fingers on the thumb side of the palmar side (underside) of the hand. The symptoms are particularly prominent at night and may awaken the patient. An examiner can reproduce the symptoms by tapping the palmar side of the patient's wrist. The initial treatment is to splint the athlete's wrist at night. If this doesn't work, I prescribe anti-inflammatory drugs and advise the patient to wear the splint during the day and to cut back on the offending activity, such as wheelchair basketball. If pain persists, I inject the wrist with a cortisone medication. If all else fails, a surgical procedure can be performed to release the entrapped nerve.

HAND INJURIES

The hand contains nineteen major bones and numerous ligaments and muscles and is capable of many complex actions. Consequently, a wide variety of sports injuries are possible. Following are some of the most common.

A *boxer's fracture* occurs when one athlete punches another, breaking the knuckle of the fifth finger. These injuries do not occur in boxing because the combatants wear padded boxing gloves. This is a common injury in martial arts and occurs in football when a player's hand strikes an opponent's helmet. Fights that occasionally break out at sporting events may also result in this type of injury. A child with a boxer's fracture will complain of pain in the knuckle of the little finger. On examination it will seem as if the knuckle disappears when the player makes a fist. The fracture can be splinted and heals in four to six weeks.

A companion injury is the human bite, which occurs as a result of an intentional or accidental punch in the mouth by another player. This can be a very serious injury. The injury may result in a bloodborne disease or a bacterial infection. First-aid treatment is to wash the area immediately and thoroughly with soap and water and to contact your physician, who will probably begin antibiotics for all but the most superficial of these injuries.

Another common and potentially serious injury is the *skier's thumb* (Fig. 13). It occurs when a skier's thumb is caught on the ski pole and the thumb is forcefully pushed away from the hand. This causes a sprained ligament with or without an associated fracture. Depending on the exact type of injury, it can sometimes

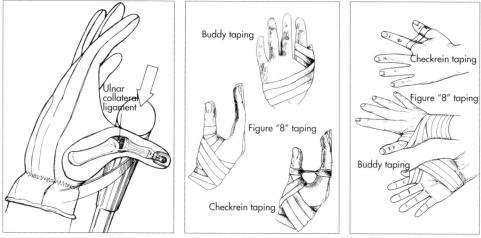

FIGURE 13 SKIER'S THUMB

be casted but may require surgery. In any case, seek medical attention for any injury to the base of the thumb. Such an injury will not heal properly unless appropriately treated. An athlete with a skier's thumb can return to competition before the injury is completely healed if the hand is taped so that the thumb cannot be forcibly pulled away from the hand (Fig. 13).

FINGER INJURIES

Finger injuries comprise 10 percent of all athletic injuries. One of the most common finger injuries is the *dislocation* of the middle knuckle. This happens when the player's finger is struck by a ball or another player. It can occur in any sport involving catching or contact. A dislocation is simply a sprain where the ligaments are stretched and one bone slides out of joint over another. The ligaments then spring back to their original position, and the bone is caught out of place (Fig. 14). This injury is often called a *coach's finger* because the coach will sometimes pull on the finger to make it go back into place (reduction). I would advise against this maneuver because in the process a piece of tissue can be caught between the bones and prevent proper reduction. Call your physician, who knows the proper technique for reducing this injury. Team physicians in attendance at a game will reduce these dislocations on the sideline and "buddy tape" the injured finger to the adjoining finger so that the athlete can return to play. Complete healing usually takes two to three weeks.

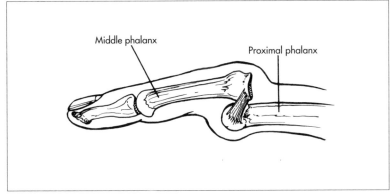

Middle phalanx

Proximal phalanx

FIGURE 14 FINGER DISLOCATION

Players often complain that they have "jammed" or "stoved" their fingers. This injury is similar to the one described above but is less severe. When the finger is jammed, the ligaments are stretched but not enough to cause the bone to dislocate. These injuries are also sprains and should be treated by buddy taping until symptoms subside.

A *baseball finger* occurs when a ball strikes the fingertip and forcibly bends it downward. This action sometimes tears the ligament and sometimes pulls off the intact ligament with a piece of bone attached (Fig. 15); the latter is called an *avulsion fracture*. In this injury the fingertip cannot be straightened by itself but can be easily straightened by someone else. This injury is easy to treat with a splint when recognized early but will lead to a permanent deformity if not properly treated. Treatment is the same of a baseball finger whether or not there is an avulsion fracture. The fingertip is immobilized in a splint in a straightened position for about six weeks. Only the end joint should be splinted. If the whole finger is splinted, unnecessary stiffness of unaffected joints will occur.

Another finger injury that occurs in sports that involve tackling is the *jersey finger*. It occurs when the finger, usually the ring finger, gets caught in an opponent's jersey as the player attempts to make a tackle. The athlete ruptures the tendon on the palmar side of the finger. Treatment is surgical.

Many of us have had the unpleasant experience of smashing a finger in a door or having it stepped on by another person, which resulted in a collection of blood beneath the fingernail. This injury is called a *subungual* (from Latin: sub—under; unguis— nail)

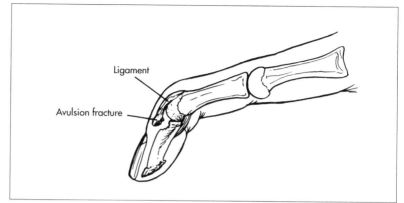

FIGURE 15 BASEBALL FINGER

hematoma (blood clot) and is extremely painful, but it is also easy to treat. Simply heat a paper clip and push it through the nail to release the collection of blood and relieve the pain. If you are fainthearted, call your physician, who can accomplish the same results with a drill in the office.

The hand is unprotected in many sports and thus subject to many sprains and bruises. The R.I.C.E. treatment (rest, ice, compression, elevation, see pp. 31–32) will cure most of them. Buddy taping the injured finger to the uninjured one next to it allows the uninjured finger to act as a splint, protecting the injured one as it moves. The taping relieves the pain of a sprain and allows players to return to competition sooner.

When a child complains of a finger injury, have him or her open the hand and then close it. Compare it with the opposite hand. Often, the injured finger will look normal when the fingers are extended but a deformity will be obvious when the patient makes a fist. If there is substantial pain, swelling, or deformity, see your doctor. Many finger injuries look insignificant at first, but if they aren't treated properly, the injury can lead to a permanent deformity with associated loss of function.

CHEST INJURIES

Serious injury from chest trauma is exceedingly rare, even in contact and collision sports. The ribs protect the heart and lungs quite well, especially in older children. A player may sustain bruised ribs or even occasionally nondisplaced rib fractures. These can be splinted with a flak jacket, and the player can return to competition as soon as comfort allows, usually in about four weeks. There is one exception to this. Younger players (six- and seven-year-olds) can suffer a bruise to the heart when struck by a ball. This can cause an irregular heart rhythm and has resulted in death. Some authorities have suggested that T-ball and Little League baseball batters wear flak jackets while batting to prevent this type of injury. Others favor a softer baseball for Little League play than is currently being used.

RESPIRATORY PROBLEMS

In addition to chest injuries, certain respiratory problems can also arise during sports activities. One of the most common is exercise-induced asthma (E.I.A.), which takes the form of wheezing that begins from five to fifteen minutes into a workout. The wheezing may not be audible even when listened to with a stethoscope, and pulmonary function tests may be necessary to make the diagnosis. The most common symptom is coughing while exercising. The athlete may also experience chest tightness and shortness of breath. As many as 10 percent of youth athletes have E.I.A. Almost all asthmatics wheeze during exercise, and about one-half of patients with respiratory allergies wheeze while exercising. Many patients don't even know that they have E.I.A., but athletes who do may complain that they get tired easily or lack stamina, particularly when exercising in the cold. Treatment is usually easy and successful once the diagnosis is made. Warming up by jogging for fifteen minutes often prevents symptoms from occurring. Inhaled medications, called bronchodilators, such as Proventil, administered twenty minutes before practice or competition, prevent symptoms in all but the severest cases. Choosing your sport can also make a big difference. Sports such as swimming, during which the respiratory system is exposed to warm, moist air, are much less likely to cause symptoms than is cross-country skiing, in which the inhaled air is cold and dry.

Another respiratory problem that we see commonly in sports is *hyperventilation*. This usually occurs in younger children who may not be in the best shape. It occurs in sports such as basketball and soccer, which require a lot of running. Players affected by hyperventilation will either leave the game or stand in the middle of the field complaining of difficulty in breathing. They may also complain of numbness or tingling in the fingertips or around the mouth. The symptoms are caused by the fact that these children are breathing too fast and, in so doing, blow off too much of the carbon dioxide in their blood when they exhale. Treatment consists of having the player breathe into a paper bag, which enables him or her to rebreathe the exhaled carbon dioxide. After a minute or two, the symptoms will go away. The child can resume practice or play immediately after symptoms subside.

Influenza, a viral respiratory infection that affects both athletes and nonathletes during the winter months, causes symptoms that may prevent an athlete from competing for a week or two but rarely causes significant problems in healthy individuals. Young athletes with chronic medical problems (e.g., diabetes or asthma), however, can have serious problems if they contract the flu. I recommend a yearly flu shot for these children.

Injuries of the Abdomen, Genitals, and Back

ABDOMINAL INJURIES

Unlike the chest, the abdominal organs have no external bony protection. Blunt trauma to the abdomen can cause severe injury. The most common serious injury is a ruptured *spleen*. The spleen is located in the upper abdomen just under the lower ribs on the left side. When it is ruptured, the athlete will complain of pain in that area, particularly when firm pressure is applied during a medical examination. The patient may have pain with inhaling. In severe cases, when the spleen is ruptured, evidence of shock as a result of internal bleeding will be seen. These signs are light-headedness, sweating, and a rapid pulse.

THE MOST COMMON SERIOUS INJURY IS A RUPTURED SPLEEN.

Parents and coaches should all be aware of this potentially life-threatening injury. Always consider the possibility of a splenic rupture when a player complains of lower left rib pain, and call 911 if there is any suspicion of this injury.

Because the spleen is an organ that plays an important role in preventing infections, we try to avoid its surgical removal whenever possible. Patients with a ruptured spleen but no evidence of internal bleeding can be admitted to the hospital and observed for a period of about one week. If they are stable at the end of this time, surgery is avoided and they can be discharged. But these patients cannot return to contact sports until the CAT scan has returned to normal. This process often takes a few months. If the spleen does have to be surgically removed, the athlete should receive a Pneumovax immunization. This will help prevent some of the infections that the spleen protected against. One vaccination may be good for a lifetime of protection.

Infectious mononucleosis is a condition that causes an enlarged spleen and makes it more susceptible to rupture, even after relatively minor trauma. Mono, as it is more commonly called, most often affects teenagers. It is also referred to as "the kissing disease" because it is caused by close personal contact such as kissing or sharing drinks from bottles or cans. It tends to be epidemic. When I see an athlete with mono, I withhold him from sports for four weeks from the onset of the illness, even if the spleen appears to be normal size in physical exam. If the spleen is enlarged upon examination, I keep the player out of practice until the organ returns to normal size, which is determined by ultrasound examination.

TESTICULAR INJURIES

Testicular injuries should be rare in sports. Boys playing contact sports should be required to wear plastic protective cups. Any boy with an injured or congenitally absent testicle should likewise wear a cup to protect the remaining uninjured testicle, even if he is participating in a sport that usually doesn't result in contact or collisions. If a boy is struck in the testicle and is not wearing a cup, the most likely injury that he will sustain is a bruise. This injury may be very painful at first, but the severe pain should subside within a few minutes. If severe pain persists, consult your physician, who will then order an ultrasound to rule out more serious injuries such as a ruptured or twisted testicle. The latter injury requires surgical correction within about six hours to save the testicle. This injury is most common among boys aged eleven to thirteen.

BACK INJURIES

Most of us will hurt our backs at one time or another during our lifetimes. The most common injuries are muscle strains and ligament sprains, caused by stretching muscles and ligaments beyond the range of motion that they were intended for. These injuries occur as a result of heavy lifting or twisting. We used to put athletes to bed, often in traction, to treat these injuries. Studies demonstrate that this treatment actually prolongs the athlete's recovery rather than hastens it. Treatment now consists of relative rest, during which the patient avoids those activities that are painful and performs other activities to tolerance. Most athletes can return to competition in a couple of weeks.

Hamstring (the large muscle group in the back of the thigh) *tightness* predisposes a person to back injuries, but they can be prevented by promoting hamstring flexibility. This involves performing specific stretching exercises such as toe touches or hurdler's exercises (Fig. 16).

Kidney trauma occurs as a result of a blow to the back above the waist. This trauma can result in anything from a contusion to

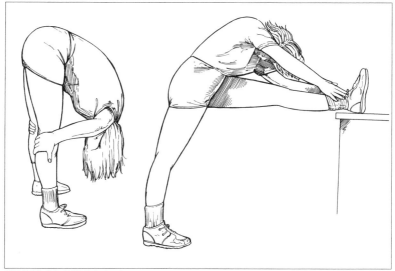

FIGURE 16 EXERCISES FOR HAMSTRING FLEXIBILITY

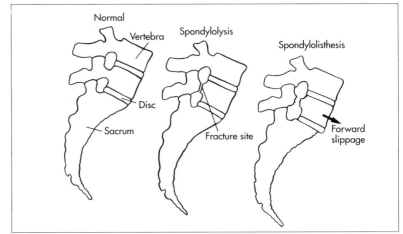

FIGURE 17 SPONDYLOLYSIS: STRESS FRACTURE OF THE SPINE

a rupture of the kidney. If an athlete complains of back pain and a dusky discoloration or actual blood in the urine, seek immediate medical attention. The physician will order an x-ray or other imaging study to determine whether the kidney is simply bruised or whether a more serious injury has occurred. Most cases of kidney trauma will necessitate avoidance of participation until the injury resolves; more severe injury may require surgery.

Spondylolysis and *spondylolisthesis* are back injuries that commonly occur in adolescents. Spondylolysis is a stress fracture of the spine resulting from overuse (Fig. 17). Spondylolisthesis is a slippage of one vertebra over another as a result of a stress fracture that occurs on both sides of the same vertebra. Spondylolysis occurs in 6 percent of the general population, partly as a result of heredity and partly from the activities that the teen performs. Divers who arch their backs frequently as part of their sport have about a 63 percent incidence of spondylolysis. Weight lifters, wrestlers, and gymnasts have an incidence of 30 to 35 percent, and spondylolysis occurs in 15 to 25 percent of track and field athletes and football players. These problems are commonly associated with the adolescent growth spurt. If your son or daughter has back pain, particularly if he or she participates in any of these sports, you can often make a tentative diagnosis yourself. If your child has pain that persists more than two weeks, it is more likely due to spondylolysis than to a sprain or strain.

I use a test called the "wall slide" test, which I believe is very reliable in diagnosing this condition. To perform this test have

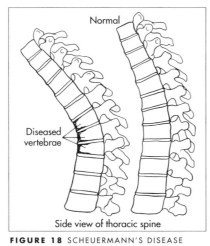

Normal

Diseased vertebrae

Side view of thoracic spine

FIGURE 18 SCHEUERMANN'S DISEASE

your child stand with his back against a wall and bend the knees and hips so as to slide down the wall. If he has pain with this maneuver, he probably has either spondylolysis or spondylolisthesis and should see a sports medicine physician. If there is a minimal degree of slippage and the athlete has symptoms, relative rest is all that is needed. When the athlete is pain-free he or she may return to competition. If there is a significant degree of slippage of one vertebra over the vertebra below, bracing and even surgery may be necessary in more serious situations.

Scheuermann's disease is another malady affecting the spine that occurs in adolescents. Although it is not a sports injury, I include it here because I have seen several patients with this problem who erroneously thought they had injured themselves while playing sports. The patients have pain in the upper back, roughly between the shoulder blades. The pain can be severe. The diagnosis is made by taking x-rays of the upper spine, which show an area that appears to be missing from the vertebrae (Fig. 18). Treatment consists of avoiding activities that cause pain. Bracing the spine is necessary in severe cases.

Leg Injuries

HIP INJURIES

Serious hip injuries are distinctly unlikely in youth sports. There are two problems, both associated with growth and development, that can affect youth sports participation. The first of these is *Legg-Calve-Perthes disease*. This is a problem that affects children, with the peak incidence occurring at approximately five years of age. It is caused by a hip socket that is too shallow, allowing the hip to dislocate or pop out of joint. It is not a sports injury, strictly speaking, but I mention it because parents of children who complain of persistent pain with activity should not

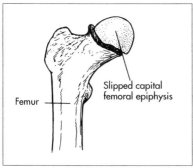

FIGURE 19 HIP INJURIES

Slipped capital femoral epiphysis

Femur

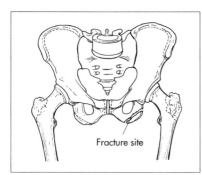

FIGURE 20 GROWTH PLATE

Fracture site

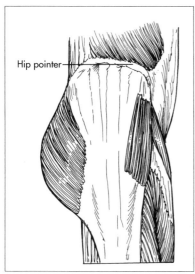

FIGURE 21 HIP POINTER

Hip pointer

simply dismiss their complaints as sore muscles. A child who complains of persistent pain should be evaluated. The second problem is a *slipped capital femoral epiphysis,* which presents similarly but occurs in adolescents. This is a disruption of the growth plate in which the ball of the hip joint slips off the bone (Fig. 19).

Again, my recommendation is to seek medical attention when a young athlete complains of persistent pain in the leg, whether or not the cause of the pain is a traumatic injury. It is important to note that both of these conditions cause a dull pain, which is most noticeable in the knee rather than the hip and is often accompanied by a limp. Both of these conditions occur much more often in boys than in girls and may manifest themselves after an insignificant sports injury. Taking an x-ray of the affected hip will provide the definitive diagnosis. The former disease is usually treated by bracing, the latter by surgical correction.

The *growth plate,* or *epiphysis,* of a bone is an area of cartilage between two sections of bone where growth occurs (Fig. 20). It is weaker than the surrounding bone and therefore subject to injury. Typically, the growing part of the bone is pulled away from the rest of the bone as a result of violent muscle contraction. If the separation is less than a quarter inch, the fracture will heal with a few weeks' rest. When the separation is more than a quarter inch, surgery is usually required to reattach the fractured fragment. Growth plate injuries rarely occur in younger children because they don't have the muscle mass to cause sufficient force to produce these types of injuries. They don't occur in adults because the growth plates close and disappear when we're finished growing. Growth plate injuries are common in adolescents.

Another hip injury is the *hip pointer,* a contusion or strain or even a fracture at the site where abdominal muscles insert on the hip (Fig. 21). It occurs when a blow to the torso either bruises the muscle or bends the upper body away and stretches the muscles. This injury will usually take two or three weeks to heal. If a player plays with this type of injury, there is some discomfort but no risk of causing a long-term problem. Hip pointers are often caused by ill-fitting hip pads worn by football players. Make sure that your children go off to practice with properly fitting equipment.

THIGH INJURIES

There are several acute injuries to the *thigh* (upper leg) that are common in sports. These are strains of the *groin muscles, hamstrings,* and *quadriceps.* These injuries are a result not of contact or collisions but of forcibly overstretching these muscles. The groin muscles are on the medial aspect (inside) of the upper leg. They flex the hip and pull the leg toward the middle of the body. These muscles can be injured when an athlete changes direction while running. The injury occurs to the leg that is planted when the thigh is forcibly abducted (pulled away from the body). The hamstring, the muscle group in the back of the thigh, is pulled or strained as a result of forcibly pushing off while sprinting. The incidence of these injuries can be reduced by warming up and stretching before competing. These muscle strains take a few weeks to heal and are often aggravated if a player continues to compete before he or she is completely healed. Most players do continue to play with this type of injury after the acute phase and don't heal completely until after their season is finished. No permanent or serious damage occurs as a result of playing with these types of injuries.

The quadriceps muscles are the large muscle group in the front of the thigh. The quadriceps are often injured in contact sports when the thigh is struck by an opponent's helmet or shoulder pads. To protect against this injury, in football, a sport in which quad contusions are very common because of the amount of contact, the player wears thigh pads. These contusions are also common soccer injuries as a result of collisions between players at the time one player is attempting to kick the ball. Quadriceps injuries have been estimated as comprising 10 percent of all athletic injuries. If a quadriceps contusion is recognized early, recovery will progress faster. Most parents underestimate the seriousness of this type of injury. If your child is limping and complains of pain in the front of the thigh, he or she has probably sus-

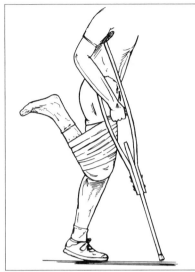

FIGURE 22 SPLINT FOR QUADRICEPS CONTUSION

tained a quadriceps contusion. Call your physician. In cases of a severe injury the sports medicine physician will splint the leg in a flexed position for a day or two (Fig. 22), while the injured player gets around with the aid of crutches. After this, the player may bear weight without crutches and begin isometric exercises. When the child can walk without pain, he or she begins range-of-motion and strengthening exercises before returning to competition.

Another problem of the upper leg is *femoral anteversion.* This is not an injury but rather a congenital condition in which the feet "toe in" because the upper leg is twisted inward. This situation usually corrects itself, at least partially, by age eight. It is not a contraindication to sports participation. In fact, I look at it as a variation of normal. We used to treat this problem with bracing and special shoes. We no longer do this because treatment is ineffective.

KNEE INJURIES

The knee is a complex structure stabilized on the inside and outside of the joint by the medial and lateral collateral ligaments, respectively, which prevent the knee from collapsing side to side. Within the joint itself there are the anterior and posterior cruciate ligaments (*cruciate* means cross-shaped), which add stability in the forward and backward direction. These structures cross within the joint space. There are also two half-moon-shaped cartilages that further stabilize the joint (Fig. 23). Any of these structures can be injured when torsional or twisting forces are applied to the joint.

The knee is the site of many serious injuries. Several promising careers have been shortened when an athlete "blew out a knee." We use this terminology when we are referring to a *complete tear* (third-degree sprain) of the athlete's *anterior cruciate ligament (ACL)* (Fig. 24).

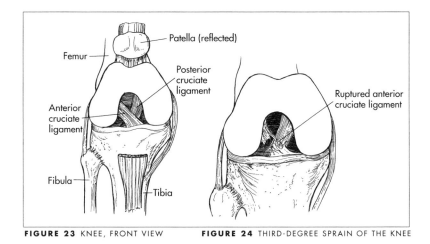

FIGURE 23 KNEE, FRONT VIEW   **FIGURE 24** THIRD-DEGREE SPRAIN OF THE KNEE

The athlete experiences pain and a feeling that the knee has given way. He or she may say that he or she felt a pop and noted immediate swelling. The physical examination of these athletes is sometimes confusing, especially if they have very muscular thighs. The definitive diagnosis can be made with MRI. Most experts will wait four to six weeks after the acute injury to reconstruct the ACL. In the skeletally mature youth with a closed growth plate, doctors can perform the surgical procedure through the laporo-scope, using a tendon graft. Up to one year of rigorous rehabilita-tion is often necessary before a return to sports. This injury is often associated with a tear of the *medial meniscus* and *medial collateral ligament* as well. Fortunately, I see few of these or other serious knee injuries before high school age.

An athlete can sprain the medial collateral ligament when another player lands on the outside of the knee, collapsing it toward the inside. I x-ray the knee of a young teen with an open growth plate who is injured in this way more often than I do the knee of an adult or skeletally mature teen. The growth plate (epi-physis) is a relatively weak structure and may be fractured in what looks otherwise like a minor sprain. An unrecognized fracture in a growth plate can lead to problems as the bone grows. The growth plate of the distal femur (the part of the long bone in the thigh nearest the knee) begins to fuse at age thirteen in girls and age fifteen in boys. After this time they are skeletally mature in this area, and x-rays are less important in evaluating sprains.

The knee is often injured in sports when the foot is planted and the upper leg is twisted. This can happen simply while changing direction during running, but it often occurs when a player is blocked with his or her foot planted. The football rule makers have appropriately outlawed "clipping," blocking from behind the midpoint of the body, because this is a major cause of serious knee injuries. It is important for coaches to stress proper blocking technique; fewer injuries will result.

The *meniscus,* or *semilunar cartilage,* is, as the name implies, a half-moon or C-shaped structure on the inner and outer aspect of the knee. The medial meniscus is injured three times as often as the lateral meniscus. Injury occurs as a result of twisting forces. The injured person complains of pain and a history of the joint's locking. Upon physical examination there is tenderness along the medial joint line, minimal swelling, and a painful click when the flexed knee is extended and simultaneously twisted. Often the knee can't be fully extended because the cartilage is caught in the joint space between the bones. Smaller tears require no treatment except rest, ice, and anti-inflammatory medications. If the patient continues to have pain or complains that the joint is locking, surgery is required. I like to wait about a month before I refer the patient for arthroscopic surgery. This allows time for the tear to heal on its own and for swelling to decrease. During this time, ligaments that were injured at the time of the meniscus injury can also heal.

Another acute knee injury is the *hyperextended knee.* This injury occurs in contact and collision sports when a player is hit in the leg with the knee straight. The athlete complains of pain in the back of the knee because the ligaments in that area are stretched at the time of the injury. He or she may also complain of pain in the front of the joint below the knee because the leg bone is compressed at the time of contact. This injury is usually not serious and the player can be treated with R.I.C.E. and return to action in two to three weeks. However, there are two situations that can turn this minor injury into a major one. First, the knee can temporarily dislocate, injuring the blood vessels in the back of the leg. Second, the force of the blow can cause the ACL to pull off a section of bone. To detect these serious complications, always check the pulse in the back of the knee when a player comes off the field after hyperextending his knee, and always get an x-ray in any hypertension injuries that are more than minor injuries.

In a high school or college sporting event, one will see that many players have their knees protected with some type of knee

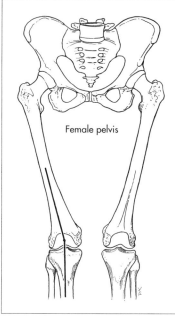

FIGURE 25 SLANT OF UPPER LEG
BONES IN WOMEN

Female pelvis

brace. These are prescribed by the team physician on an individual basis to protect a knee that has been previously injured. There is no controversy regarding their use. There is controversy, however, over another use of the knee brace that has been prescribed to protect a normal knee against injury. Many experts believe these preventive braces protect against injuries caused by twisting the knee; others believe either that the braces are of no value or that wearing them may even cause an increased risk of injury to the knee.

The knee is also subject to chronic overuse injuries. A common one is *patello-femoral stress syndrome,* which refers to pain caused by a partial dislocation of the knee, called *subluxation,* that occurs during running. The cause of this condition is an uneven pull on the knee cap toward the outside of the leg when the knee is bent and straightened. It happens because of weakness in the large muscle group on the front of the thigh, particularly the muscle on the innermost aspect of the quadriceps group called the *vastus medialis oblique* (VMO). This condition is most prevalent in adolescent female runners. Women have a wider pelvis than men to facilitate childbearing, so the upper legs slant toward the middle of the body as the bone approaches the knee, causing an exaggeration of the lateral pull described above (Fig. 25). This anatomical alignment causes the increased incidence of injury. Treatment consists of simple exercises to strengthen the muscle in question (Fig. 26) and ibuprofen for pain and inflammation. The patient should scale back his or her exercise program until the discomfort subsides. Some physicians, including me, prescribe an inexpensive neoprene knee brace with a hole cut out for the kneecap, which can be purchased at a sporting goods store. The brace is thought to warm the joint during exercise, which lessens discomfort. It may also help with patellar alignment during

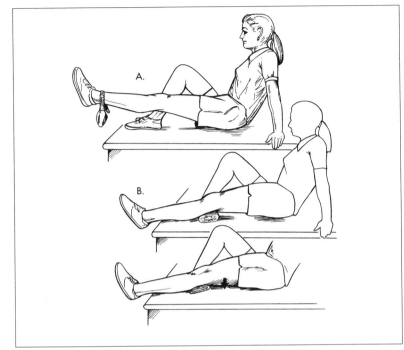

FIGURE 26 EXERCISES FOR PATELLO-FEMORAL STRESS SYNDROME

flexion (bending) and extension (straightening) of the knee.

Another overuse injury of the knee has the exotic name *iliotibial band syndrome (ITB),* which is a type of tendinitis. This injury occurs because the band (which is a tendon) causes friction as it passes over the outside of the knee joint when the knee is repeatedly bent and straightened during running (Fig. 27).

It is very common in running sports and produces pain on the outside of the runner's knee. It typically comes at the same time or distance in the training run. The athlete describes a burning pain that occurs during the landing phase of the gait when the foot strikes the ground. On physical examination there is a tender point on the outside of the knee but no pain on motion of the knee. The injury usually occurs on the downhill knee (the left, if the runner trains facing the oncoming traffic) in runners who train by running along the side of the road. ITB is treated like most overuse injuries, with R.I.C.E. and stretching (Fig. 28).

Osgood-Schlatter syndrome is a knee problem unique to children twelve to fifteen years old. It is caused by pulling on the structures around the growth plate just below the knee. The children may

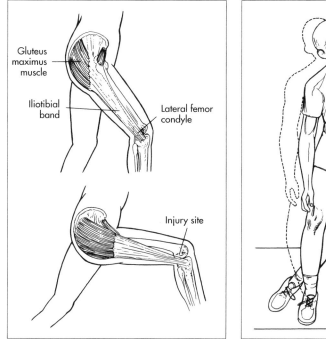

Gluteus
maximus
muscle

Iliotibial
band

Lateral femor
condyle

Injury site

FIGURE 27 ILIOTIBIAL BAND SYNDROME

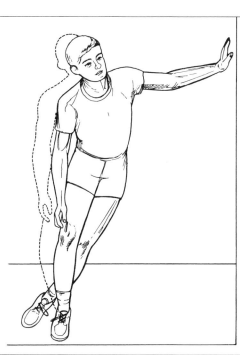

FIGURE 28 STRETCHING EXERCISE FOR ILIOTIBIAL
BAND SYNDROME

experience a growth spurt at this age, and the ligaments just can't
keep up. Children with this condition experience pain and a tender
bump below the knee. The pain is aggravated by weight-bearing
activity. X-rays of the leg should be taken to rule out a more serious
problem. Treatment is to cut back on activity until the discomfort
resolves. The bump may remain, but if the pain is gone, the patient
may participate in sports without restriction.

Jumper's knee, or *patellar tendinitis,* is an injury of the
ligament below the kneecap. Patients complain of pain below the
kneecap that occurs after running or jumping. Jumper's knee is an
overuse injury and occurs primarily in jumping sports such as basketball, volleyball, ballet, and gymnastics. The treatment is
relative rest and anti-inflammatory agents such as ibuprofen.

Shin splints is a term familiar to cross-country and track athletes. It refers to lower leg (technically, the lower leg is the *leg,* and upper leg is the *thigh*) pain, which includes several different diagnoses. Shin pain often occurs on the inside aspect of the front of the lower leg. It is caused by inflammation of the covering of the bone at the point where a tendon attaches. Typically the pain initially comes on after running. Next it occurs during, as well as after, the run, and, if the injury is severe enough, it can also occur at rest. If the athlete persists in rigorous training, the result can be a stress fracture of the lower leg bone.

AS WITH MOST OVERUSE INJURIES, THE BEST TREATMENT IS PREVENTION.

A *stress fracture* is an actual break in the bone caused by repeated microtrauma rather than one violent traumatic event. Stress fractures account for about 10 percent of all athletic injuries. The vast majority of them are of the lower extremities because the legs are subject to both overuse and the effects of weight bearing. The tibia (the larger bone in the lower leg) is the most common site for stress fractures, accounting for almost half the total number. Stress fractures result from overtraining and typically occur when an athlete increases either the frequency, speed, or distance of the workouts. This often happens when an athlete is trying to get in shape during the preseason. They can also be triggered by a change in training surface (e.g., going from a dirt path to a concrete roadway), by wearing running shoes that are worn out and have lost their resiliency, or by an abnormality in the child's stride, such as overpronating (pronation is a condition in which the ankle rolls over the foot toward the middle after the landing phase of the gait). Poor mechanics are also contributory, and a sports medicine physician can often correct this problem.

The diagnosis of a stress fracture is based on a high index of clinical suspicion. X-rays are often negative at first and don't become positive for the stress fracture until three weeks after the injury. If your child has pain, especially in the setting of the risk factors just discussed, the sports medicine physician will order a bone scan to make the diagnosis. MRI is a useful tool to diagnose stress fracture, but I rarely use it because it is expensive (approximately $1500).

As with most overuse injuries, the best treatment is prevention. The best way to avoid these problems is to increase gradually the athlete's workload. I recommend increasing the distance run by no more than 10 percent every two weeks and when possible varying the type of training. For example, distance runners could train by running long distances slowly on Monday and Thursday, running shorter distances at a pace one minute per mile slower than their race pace on Tuesday and Friday, running sprints on Wednesday, and competing on Saturday. Adolescent females, especially those who are very thin and are not menstruating, are particularly vulnerable to stress fractures. These girls need calcium supplements and sometimes estrogen replacement.

When stress fractures occur, however, the treatment is relative rest. This means avoiding the activities that cause pain until the symptoms abate but continuing a normal daily nonsport routine. For example, this usually requires refraining from track practice but rarely requires that the athlete use crutches or casting. During the time the athletes are not practicing, they should perform other exercises, such as swimming or cycling, in order to maintain the level of cardiovascular fitness required in their sports. When the pain goes away they can begin flexibility exercises and weight training. Only after this step should they resume practice for their specific sports.

I tell athletes to practice every other day at first. If they participate in running sports, I have them jog for a week and then run at one minute per mile slower than their usual training pace for another two weeks. Runners can then train and race at their usual pace if they remain pain-free. I usually keep high school runners training on an every-other-day schedule for the rest of that season. I often prescribe orthotics (arch supports) if the runner's stride suffers from a biomechanical problem that causes overpronating.

When our kids play as youngsters, they rarely experience these overuse injuries. When they get tired, they stop playing. As older youths, either because of the addition of coaches and a higher level of competition, or simply because of the adolescent's desire to excel, they often overtrain and injure themselves.

Medial tibial stress syndrome is a condition that involves the lower leg and can often be confused with stress fracture. These two overuse injuries differ in that a stress fracture involves tenderness at a certain point, whereas the medial tibial stress syndrome patient experiences more diffuse pain. If the athlete can point with one finger to the place that hurts, it is a stress fracture. Athletes with medial tibial stress syndrome have pain earlier during the training run and the pain goes away as they continue running; the opposite is true of athletes with a stress fracture.

A compartment syndrome is another type of lower leg injury. This occurs when the muscle is simply too big for the surrounding tissue that encloses it. The muscle in the athlete hypertrophies or enlarges, but the surrounding tissue can't. When the athlete is running, the leg also fills up with blood, which makes it even larger with respect to the enclosing tissue. Compartment syndromes can be either acute or chronic. An acute compartment syndrome is a medical emergency. The player will complain of pain in the leg that worsens with time. On examination the leg is swollen and tender. Movement of the ankle often makes the pain worse. If your child has these symptoms after an athletic contest or practice, elevate and ice the leg. If symptoms don't resolve in one hour, call your physician. If an acute compartment syndrome is diagnosed, emergency surgery to split the overlying tissue is required. Chronic compartment syndrome symptoms are less dramatic. Leg pain usually occurs during training or competition but is relieved by rest. However, each time the athlete trains, the symptoms can recur. Surgical release of the tissue around the muscle is the treatment of choice for this condition, but on an elective rather than emergency basis.

Muscle cramps are a very common athletic occurrence, but they rarely require attention from the physician. Most of the ones I see are in the calf muscle. They are very common among athletes who wear anything that constricts their calves, including knee braces. No one is exactly sure why athletes suffer from muscle cramps. There seems to be a consensus that certain athletes have a lot of cramps and others never do. Because cramps are most common in hot weather, most of us involved in sports medicine believe that athletes cramp because of dehydration or a loss of chemicals called electrolytes in the perspiration. I believe that the incidence of cramps can be lessened by keeping the athletes well hydrated with an electrolyte-containing drink like Gatorade. Treatment is simple and effective. If a cramp occurs, simply stretch the involved muscle. For example, if the calf muscle cramps, flex the ankle by grasping the foot and bending it up toward the athlete's head to stretch the muscle. Massaging the muscle also works.

Though muscle strains and bruises are more common injuries, in my practice the injury that brings the largest number of young athletes to seek medical attention is the ankle sprain. Ankle sprains (Fig. 29) are injuries to the ligaments that stabilize the ankle (Fig. 30). They most frequently occur when the ankle is inverted or turned in. This often happens when a basketball player jumps and lands on another player's foot. The player experiences pain on the outside of the ankle joint. Treatment is the standard R.I.C.E. protocol along with ibuprofen or acetaminophen for pain. It is important to rehabilitate the ankle properly to ensure healing and prompt return to participation. It should be iced for the first forty-eight hours. We used to tell the injured athlete not to bear weight on the injured ankle, but now we encourage early weight bearing to tolerance, as this promotes faster healing.

One of the primary goals of treatment is to prevent recurrent sprains. An injured ankle becomes susceptible to recurrent injury for two reasons. First, the ankle ligaments are a sling that prevent the foot from turning inward when a person lands incorrectly. Once they are stretched as a result of a sprain, the sling becomes looser. The injured ankle should be immobilized in an Aircast for about two weeks, depending on the severity of the injury. This tightens the structures, lessening the likelihood of reinjury. The Aircast allows for flexion of the ankle up and down but prevents bending inward or outward. Second, an ankle sprain damages nerves, making it impossible for a person to feel where the foot is when it is put down. I prescribe proprioception and strengthening exercises to remedy this condition (Fig. 31).

These exercises are similar to the ones prescribed for stroke patients; they retrain the nerves and muscles so that one can feel

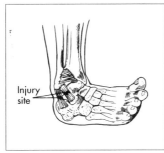

FIGURE 29 ANKLE SPRAIN

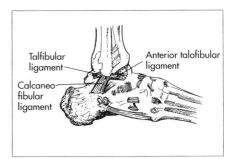

FIGURE 30 ANKLE LIGAMENTS

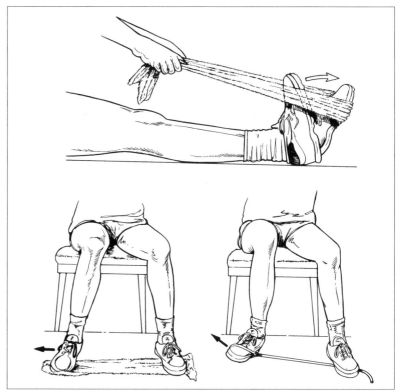

FIGURE 31 EXERCISES FOR A SPRAINED ANKLE

where the ankle is without looking down and can put the foot down flat on the ground rather than on its side, causing ankle reinjury. Ankle sprains, like any other ligament sprains, are graded one through three according to severity, with grade three being a complete tear. Surgery used to be common for the grade-three injuries, but now we treat all types of ankle sprains conservatively.

FOOT INJURIES

The foot, like the hand, is a very complex structure. It is subject to overuse stress fractures because it is weight-bearing. The location of a particular fracture is somewhat sport-specific. For example, basketball players tend to fracture the fifth metatarsal bone on the far outside of the foot as a result of the repeated jumping involved in their sport.

Severs syndrome, an overuse injury of the foot, is unique to the pediatric population (Fig. 32). It is similar to Osgood Schlatter

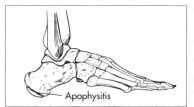

FIGURE 32 SEVERS SYNDROME

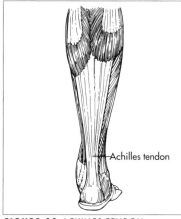

FIGURE 33 ACHILLES TENDON WITH INFLAMMATION

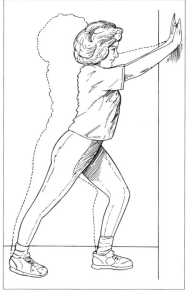

FIGURE 34 EXERCISES FOR ACHILLES TENDINITIS

syndrome but affects the heel rather than the knee and typically occurs in eleven-year-olds rather than in teenagers. It is an inflammatory problem of the growth plate and disappears when the growth plate closes. Severs syndrome is aggravated by activity such as running and improved by rest. Often it occurs in children who play multiple sports during one season or those who play in more than one league. I treat this condition with rubber heel cups, stretching exercises, ice, and reduction in activity. In my experience it is easier to treat Severs syndrome than Osgood Schlatter syndrome because the children are younger and are more likely to follow instructions to cut back on their activity level.

Achilles tendinitis is an overuse injury affecting the tendon that inserts on the back of the heel (Fig. 33). I see this mostly in older athletes, but I have occasionally seen it in teenage runners who have increased the pace or distance of their training runs. The runner has pain in the Achilles tendon where it inserts on the heel. Treatment includes stretching (Fig. 34), ice, heel cups, and anti-inflammatory medication. Runners should avoid running up hills until they are asymptomatic. Achilles tendinitis should never be treated with cortisone injections, since this can lead to tendon rupture.

Pump bumps is another condition affecting the foot. The name refers to a lump on the back of the foot just above the heel. The condition affects teenage girls and is thought to be related to wearing shoes that rub the heel at the point of contact in a patient who has a prominent heel. It is manifested by pain and swelling of the heel and can be avoided or treated by wearing appropriately fitting shoes. If this treatment fails, heel lifts similar to those used in Severs syndrome may be helpful.

Plantar faciitis is an inflammatory overuse injury of the tissue on the bottom of the foot that runs from the front of the heel to an area just

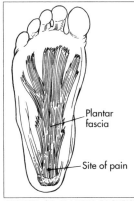

Plantar fascia

Site of pain

FIGURE 35 PLANTAR FACIITIS

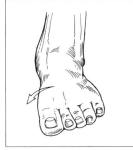

FIGURE 36 PRONATED (FLAT) FOOT

behind where the toes join the foot. The athlete experiences pain on the front inside of the heel (Fig. 35). Pain is worse when he or she gets out of bed in the morning and improves as the child walks around. Athletes will typically have pain while standing, which goes away when they are sitting. Treatment includes stretching, arch supports, ice, anti-inflammatory medicine, and cortisone injections. Some sports medicine experts prescribe night braces to hold the ankle flexed, which makes sense, but the braces are expensive and other treatments are equally effective.

Many of the chronic overuse injuries that affect the leg and foot are a result of overpronating, a condition related to flat feet. Though the patient may appear to have an adequate arch while sitting, he or she may pronate excessively when standing. This can be diagnosed by having the child stand facing away from the examiner. If the ankles seem to roll to the middle rather than remain positioned directly above the heel, the child is probably overpronating (Fig. 36 depicts pronation).

If overuse injuries to the leg, ankle, or foot are seen in the presence of this anatomic abnormality, consult a sports medicine podiatrist or physician. Orthotics (supports) are frequently prescribed to correct this condition. I prefer the inexpensive CAPI or Spenco longitudinal arch supports to the rigid and expensive plastic or leather orthotics as initial treatment. I advise the athlete to remove the insole of the running shoe and replace it with the arch support.

No sports medicine book would be complete without a section on athletic shoes. Many foot and leg injuries in runners can be prevented by wearing properly fitting shoes and changing them often. I recommend getting new running shoes after every six months or 500 miles, even if they don't show signs of wear. The problem is that despite advances in the design and manufacture of sports shoes, the midsole wears out after that distance. Wearing shoes with an air cushion in the midsole may prolong shoe life. Athletes with high-arched feet should wear curved-sole shoes with greater cushioning; those with flat feet should wear straight-sole shoes with more control. To determine whether a young athlete has a flat foot or a high-arched foot, have him or her walk in the sand. If you can see the whole outline of the foot, the child is flat-footed. If you can see only an imprint of the ball and heel of the foot, the child has a high-arched foot.

Skin Injuries

CONTUSIONS, LACERATIONS, AND BLOODBORNE DISEASES

Many athletic injuries affect the skin. Additionally, many skin conditions resulting from infections, not injuries, affect sports participation. Lacerations (cuts) and contusions (bruises) are the most common skin injuries. Contusions are treated with rest and ice and are usually self-limiting. Because of concern of transmitting *acquired immunodeficiency syndrome (AIDS)* through mixing of athletes' blood during a sporting event, the treatment of lacerations has taken on heightened priority in sports medicine in the nineties. I typically treat lacerations by suturing them on the sideline and letting the athlete return to play if the injury is not serious. However, many sports medicine physicians and trainers use superglue to close superficial lacerations. There is some recent evidence in the sports medicine literature that sutured lacerations heal faster than those closed with superglue.

ANYONE WHO IS KNOWN TO BE HIV POSITIVE SHOULD BE PROHIBITED FROM PLAYING CONTACT AND COLLISION SPORTS.

However, if a physician is not immediately available to suture the laceration and the injury is a superficial one and will not be a cosmetic problem, superglue can be a good alternative. In this era of concern over bloodborne infections such as AIDS and *hepatitis B,* it makes much more sense to allow the trainer to close the laceration with superglue than to allow a participant to return to competition while bleeding or to prohibit him or her from competing at all.

With regard to the topic of lacerations in sports, I would like to address what I see as hypocrisy on the part of the medical community regarding the transmission of bloodborne infections such as AIDS and hepatitis B. I think that we are being irresponsible in our position on the transmission of human immunodeficiency virus (HIV) or AIDS and other diseases through mixing of blood and body fluids as a result of sports injuries. This type of transmission can occur when, for example, a basketball player elbows another in the mouth. The first player sustains a laceration of the elbow as a result of the contact, and the second loosens a tooth; the blood of the players is commingled because of the injury. We insist with great confidence that the likelihood of contracting HIV through an injury like this is remote. Furthermore, there has never been a documented case of HIV transmitted as a result of an athletic injury. The National Basketball Association permitted Magic Johnson to play basketball despite his HIV-positive status. On the other hand, every high school basketball team carries something called "blood jerseys" that a player must change into when he or she has evidence of blood on the uniform. When a player sustains even the most trivial of injuries, he or she is greeted on the sidelines by a team physician wearing latex gloves!

We sports medicine physicians and trainers seem to be sending a mixed message: one, that HIV transmission through athletic contact never happens, and two, don't get near me or the other players with your bloody nose because we're afraid of exposure to the AIDS virus. So what are the facts? What should we advise our patients about the risk of transmitting AIDS through the types of injuries that can occur in sports?

Transmission of these bloodborne diseases is unlikely. Though no case of AIDS transmission through contact in sports has been absolutely documented, it is important to remember that AIDS is a fatal disease and there is no cure available at this time. I have never heard of tuberculosis being transmitted through sports competition, but my common sense tells me that I should prohibit any child with active tuberculosis from competing in contact and collision sports. Though this strategy may infringe on the rights of the individual to a degree, it protects a large number of participants from possibly contracting a fatal disease. I'm not saying that there should be mandatory AIDS testing before a player can participate in Little League baseball, but I do believe that anyone who is known to be HIV positive should be prohibited from playing contact and collision sports.

Hepatitis B is three hundred times more transmissible than HIV. It is transmitted the same way as HIV, through blood mixing. All children should be immunized against this disease.

BLISTERS

Blisters are another common skin condition. At first blush, they don't seem particularly debilitating, but don't tell that to a high school cross-country runner. Blisters can be prevented by wearing properly fitting shoes and two pairs of socks. Socks made of synthetic material such as polypropylene, which wick moisture away from the skin, are now recommended over cotton socks. Some athletes have a problem with excessive sweating, which predisposes them to blisters. Once I am certain that no underlying systemic illness is the cause, I prescribe Drysol for excessive perspiration. Petroleum jelly can be applied to the feet and nipples before a long run to prevent blisters. If blisters do occur, don't puncture them. The intact skin acts as a barrier to infection. As a sports physician I have treated blisters by aspirating the fluid and coating the blister with benzoin to keep the overlying skin in place. This permits competitive athletes to return to their sport, but it is painful and I wouldn't advise it for the average pediatric athlete.

BLISTERS CAN BE PREVENTED BY WEARING PROPERLY FITTING SHOES AND TWO PAIRS OF SOCKS.

WEATHER-RELATED SKIN INJURIES

Sunburn is another skin injury that occurs in sports. Obviously, children participating on the swim team outdoors in the summer are at risk; less obviously, cross-country skiers are also at risk. We now have excellent sunscreens that can prevent thermal burn. I advise a sunscreen with a skin protection factor (SPF) rating of fifteen. This means that the wearers will be subjected to the same thermal exposure wearing sunscreen as they would if they spent fifteen times as long in the sun without sunscreen. Read the label. Sunscreens containing PABA (para-aminobenzoic acid) esters are less likely to wash off in water. I recommend applying the sunscreen in the morning and again thirty minutes before competing. Certain medications in common usage are photosensitizing, which means they cause sunburn with minimal sun exposure. Tetracycline and Retin-A, which are commonly prescribed to adolescents for the treatment of acne, are photo-sensitizing agents. Check with your physician or pharmacist about any medication that your child is taking regarding its risk for photosensitivity.

Another skin condition brought on by the weather is *cold urticaria*. This is a form of hives that occurs when someone exercises in cold weather. It may be more common in people with asthma or allergies and can be treated with antihistamines such as Zyrtec. Medicines commonly used to treat ulcers, such as Tagamet, also prevent cold urticaria. The susceptible athlete should take these medications thirty minutes before he or she trains or competes in cold weather.

SKIN INFECTIONS

Children with an active *herpes virus infection* or a *bacterial skin infection* should not participate in sports such as wrestling until the infection has completely healed, because these conditions are very contagious. A herpes virus infection looks like the typical fever blister that commonly appears on lips. These fluid-filled blisters can occur anywhere on the skin, and the patient will often complain that the lesions itch or burn. I treat these infections with an antiviral medication called Zovirax, available by prescription as an ointment or a capsule. There is agreement in the medical community that an initial herpes attack can be improved by taking Zovirax. It is less clear whether recurrent herpetic infections benefit from this intervention. I believe that the herpes outbreak is at least shortened by prescribing Zovirax to be taken orally.

THERE IS AGREEMENT IN THE MEDICAL COMMUNITY THAT AN INITIAL HERPES ATTACK CAN BE IMPROVED BY TAKING ZOVIRAX.

Antibiotics are used to treat bacterial skin infections. Patients in certain sports such as wrestling must refrain from practicing and competing if they have a bacterial skin infection.

Jock itch and *athlete's foot* are both fungal infections. The former affects the groin as a reddish, itchy rash that appears on the inner thigh and, in males, typically spares the scrotum. The latter starts in the web spaces of the toes and often appears as small blisters. Both infections flourish in warm, damp conditions and thus are aggravated by hot weather and sweating. Both can be prevented by light, airy, moisture-absorbing clothing and powder. They can be effectively treated with over-the-counter antifungal preparations such as Lotrimin. If this doesn't work, consult your physician for a prescription of stronger medication either in topical form or to be taken orally.

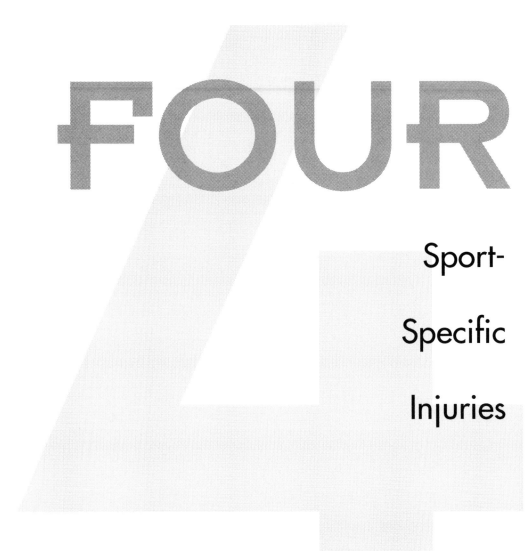

FOUR

Sport-

Specific

Injuries

CATEGORIES OF SPORTS AND INJURIES

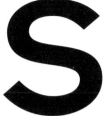

Sports can be categorized as *contact* and *collision sports, limited contact sports,* and *noncontact sports.* Noncontact sports can be divided into those that are *strenuous, moderately strenuous,* and *nonstrenuous* (see Table 1, page 6). Contact and collision sports include wrestling, lacrosse, rugby, soccer, field hockey, and football. Limited contact sports include baseball, basketball, volleyball, and gymnastics. Among noncontact sports, dance, crew, tennis, track, and swimming are examples of strenuous sports. Archery and golf are nonstrenuous. Not surprisingly, the likelihood of injury is greater in contact sports, and the types of injuries sustained are often different in each group. If any parents or coaches play golf, you already know that frustration and anxiety have nothing to do with how strenuous the sport is.

Participants in the contact and collision sports sustain injuries from collisions such as contusions, shoulder separations, and head and neck injuries. Participants in any strenuous sport are at increased risk for torque injuries such as ankle and knee sprains, and all sports participants can experience overuse injuries. Injuries can be divided into acute ones, such as an ankle sprain, and chronic injuries, such as a tennis elbow. Athletes are also subject to the same types of illness as their nonathletic peers. Some may have to stop competing because they have mononucleosis, which is an illness rather than an injury.

This part of the book discusses particular injuries in connection with the sports in which they occur most commonly. For example, tennis elbow is discussed in the section on tennis, and spondylolisthesis is discussed in the section on gymnastics. However, keep in mind that a child can rupture his or her spleen in a collision at first base as easily as when tackled playing rugby, and people can get tennis elbow from typing at a keyboard. Since most of these injuries were discussed in greater detail in part 3, this section will serve mainly as a review. *All of these injuries can benefit from R.I.C.E. therapy.*

BASEBALL

Pitching a baseball is a distinctly abnormal thing to do from a physiological perspective. It subjects the thrower's arm to a series of physical stresses. Not many people do it well. Therefore, athletes who perform this activity with skill are called upon to do it often. Pitchers are the center of attention and often become heroes. They are not likely to leave a game voluntarily, even if their arm hurts. Overuse arm injuries among young baseball players affect the shoulder and *medial aspect* of the elbow.

We hear a lot about *rotator cuff* tears among professional baseball pitchers, but younger players don't tear their rotator cuffs. Instead, youths have problems with their shoulders caused by *stress fractures* or *laxity*—also called instability of the joint—from pitching too much. These injuries can be treated by rest and rehabilitation exercises. Prevention, which means not letting the athlete pitch too often and stressing proper pitching mechanics, is always the best treatment.

YOUTHS HAVE PROBLEMS WITH THEIR SHOULDERS CAUSED BY STRESS FRACTURES OR LAXITY.

Little League elbow is a common injury to the growth plate on the medial or inside of the elbow caused by overpitching.

There have been troublesome reports of *cardiac arrests* among young baseball players who were struck in the chest by a thrown or batted ball. The mechanism postulated for these injuries is that the heart is stunned and goes into an abnormal rhythm. Players aged six and seven are susceptible because of their lack of chest muscle development and more compliant chest wall. Both of these conditions cause more of the force to be transmitted to the heart. Some experts recommend that chest protectors be worn by all participants. I don't think this is a practical solution. A more reasonable solution suggested by some is to change to a softer ball for very young players.

Other common baseball injuries are:
- **Baseball finger**—an acute injury.
  Cause: a thrown ball striking the extended finger.
  Presenting complaint: finger pain, deformity with downward flexion of the fingertip.
  Treatment: splinting the finger in an extended position.
  Surgery: occasionally necessary.
- **Carpal tunnel syndrome**—an overuse injury.
  Cause: repeatedly bending the wrist as a result of pitching.
  Presenting complaint: wrist pain and tingling in the fingertips, especially at night.
  Treatment: rest, night splint, cortisone injection.
  Surgery: occasionally necessary.

! Tips for coaches

Prevention: *Limit your pitchers to a few pitches at first, and then gradually increase the pitch count. In the typical high school season, especially in northern climates where the season is short, I would limit the pitch count to eighty, with at least four days' rest between starts. I would also have the catcher call for the "heater" 75 percent of the time. Ask your pitchers if they feel tired. Impress on them that asking to be taken out of the game is not a sign of weakness. Do not encourage young pitchers to use curve balls, and limit them with older players. If a Little Leaguer can put the ball over the plate at the knees, he'll be an All-Star. Similarly, a high school pitcher who can move the ball around doesn't need to use the breaking ball often to get batters out. The pitcher must be thoroughly warmed up before going into the game. In the middle of the summer this may take only a few minutes. In the early spring when it's cold, it may take fifteen minutes. Pitchers must throw between starts.*

The following is a workout regimen for an athlete who is a starter and pitches every six days. Day 1—pitch; day 2—off; day 3—soft toss for fifteen minutes; day 4—warm up and throw hard for twenty minutes; day 5—soft toss for fifteen minutes.

Treatment: Once a pitcher has an arm injury, be especially aware of limiting the number of pitches that he or she throws. Ice the pitcher's arm after he or she has finished pitching, no matter how few pitches have been thrown.

In addition to the injuries that basketball and volleyball players share with other competitors, they are also subject to somewhat different problems because their sport involves an inordinate amount of jumping. Not surprisingly, 75 percent of the injuries in these sports involve the lower extremity. *Jumper's knee,* or *patellar tendinitis,* is common in these athletes. It is an inflammation of the tendon below the kneecap. The athlete first has pain after competition, then during competition, and finally, pain prevents the child from competing at all. Treatment includes rest, ice, anti-inflammatory agents, and avoidance of playing on hard surfaces like concrete. *Osgood-Schlatter disease,* a knee condition, is very common in adolescent basketball and volleyball players. Other common basketball and volleyball injuries are:

- **Baseball finger**—see preceding page. This injury is more common among basketball than baseball players, since basketball players don't wear fielders' gloves.
- **Ankle sprain**—acute injury.
  Cause: landing improperly, turning the foot inward.
  Presenting complaint: pain on the outside of the ankle.
  Treatment: x-ray to rule out a fracture, R.I.C.E., immobilization.
  Surgery: rarely necessary.
- **Achilles tendinitis**—overuse injury.
  Cause: running and jumping.
  Presenting complaint: pain in the back of the heel above the heel bone associated with swelling (pain on the heel bone is more likely with Severs syndrome).
  Treatment: stretching exercises, anti-inflammatory medication.
  Surgery: Repeated episodes of tendinitis may lead to an Achilles tendon rupture, which requires either surgery or prolonged casting. This rarely occurs in children but is common in adults.
- **Fracture of fifth metatarsal**—overuse injury.
  Presenting complaint: pain on the outside of the foot.
  Treatment: cutting back on activity.
  Surgery: seldom necessary.

BOXING AND MARTIAL ARTS

Unlike professional boxing, collegiate and Golden Glove boxing work on a point system, in which body blows are rewarded as much as punches to the head. Therefore, amateur boxing is inherently safer. The bouts are also shorter at the amateur level.

Boxers and martial arts participants can suffer facial contusions and lacerations. They are subject to serious head injuries, and participants in martial arts have a disproportionate occurrence of hand and foot fractures. Martial arts competitors wear protective headgear, as well as hand and foot padding. More than half of the injuries in martial arts competition involve the head and neck. Headgear for martial arts and boxing is great for protecting against cauliflower ear and facial lacerations, but it does nothing to prevent serious injury to the brain. Despite these risks, the half million youths who participate in martial arts and boxing in this country experience an injury rate that is well below the incidence reported for basketball, football, lacrosse, or wrestling. Other common boxing and martial arts injuries are:

BOXERS AND MARTIAL ARTS PARTICIPANTS CAN SUFFER FACIAL CONTUSIONS AND LACERATIONS.

- **Concussion**—acute injury.
  Cause: blow to the head.
  Presenting complaint: confusion, amnesia, loss of consciousness.
  Treatment: withholding participant from further matches. If the athlete is unconscious, call 911: don't try to move him.
  Surgery: Boxers occasionally will develop a blood clot on the brain along with a concussion. Removal of the clot requires surgery.
- **Dementia pugalistica (punch-drunk syndrome)**—chronic injury.
  Cause: repeated blows to the head.
  Presenting complaint: confusion, slurred speech, unsteady gait.
  Treatment: prevention (giving up boxing ten years beforehand).

- **Eye trauma**—acute injury.

  Cause: striking the eye with the thumb of boxing glove.

  Presenting complaint: eye pain, visual disturbance.

  Treatment: prevention, thumbless boxing gloves. There are many different types of eye trauma, ranging from a simple hemorrhage, which can be treated by the passage of time, to a detached retina (like the one suffered by world champion Sugar Ray Leonard).

  Surgery: necessary in serious injuries like retinal detachments and fractures of the orbit.

- **Nasal fractures**—acute injuries.

  Cause: blow to the nose.

  Presenting complaint: nasal pain, bleeding.

  Treatment: ice, nasal packing if bleeding persists.

  Surgery: necessary if there is a displaced fracture.

CROSS-COUNTRY AND TRACK

These are sports that require endurance training, which means that you have to log a lot of miles to excel. Therefore, overuse injuries of the lower extremities are common. Cross-country and track athletes also suffer acute injuries, again, usually to the leg, foot, and ankle. The ankle sprain is the most common acute injury in runners. Improper equipment and differing training surfaces also contribute to overuse injuries. When a runner goes from the track to the road, training injuries often occur because the training surface is harder and less resilient. Worn running shoes also contribute to injuries. I recommend replacing the shoes every five hundred miles even if they don't show signs of wear; the shoes seem to be less resilient after they have been used for running that distance. Physical factors such as lack of flexibility and abnormal biomechanics (e.g., flat feet) are also factors in injuries to runners. Don't train by running on the same side of a crowned road all the time because this can lead to knee problems. Other cross-country and track injuries are:

> I RECOMMEND REPLACING THE SHOES EVERY FIVE HUNDRED MILES EVEN IF THEY DON'T SHOW SIGNS OF WEAR.

- **Patello-femoral stress syndrome**—overuse injury.

   Cause: overpronating while running, more common in females than in males.

   Presenting complaint: anterior knee pain, especially with climbing or descending stairs.

   Treatment: quadriceps-strengthening exercises, orthotics, neoprene knee sleeve (maybe).

   Surgery: almost never necessary.

- **Hamstring strain**—acute injury.

   Cause: rapid acceleration during the push-off phase of running.

   Presenting complaint: pain in the back of the thigh.

   Treatment: prevention (warm-up stretching exercise), R.I.C.E.

   Surgery: never.

- **Compartment syndrome**—chronic or acute.

   Cause: muscle in the leg is too big for the surrounding tissue.

   Presenting complaint: pain in the lower leg during and sometimes after running.

   Treatment: elevation of the affected leg.

   Surgery: in acute cases.

- **Plantar faciitis**—overuse injury.

   Cause: running, particularly among heavier runners.

   Presenting complaint: heel pain is worse when getting out of bed in the morning; better as the day progresses.

   Treatment: stretching, orthotics, cortisone injections.

   Surgery: occasionally necessary.

DANCE

Eating disorders and osteoporosis are common problems among dancers. Ballet rewards a lithe figure. The average young girl begins her period by about age 12$\frac{1}{2}$, but the typical ballerina doesn't start her periods until age 15$\frac{1}{2}$. Young ballerinas can sustain overuse injuries to the lower extremities. As dancers get older, they dance *en pointe*—on their toes. This puts an incredible stress on the bones of the foot connected to the first and second toes. Stress fractures of the feet are common in these bones. At first these injuries result in pain after practice. If the athlete continues to dance, the pain will occur earlier during her practice and finally will occur at rest. Treatment is to cut back on activity until symptoms subside. Taping the injured foot is sometimes helpful. These injuries occur primarily among advanced-level dancers. The vast majority of participants in youth ballet dance at the beginner's level and practice only once or twice a week; consequently, their injuries are the result of faulty technique rather than overuse. The most common problem is that they do not have the requisite flexibility, at a very young age, to execute all the basic positions required in ballet. Other dance injuries are:

- **Jumper's knee**—overuse injury.
Cause: repeated jumping.
Presenting complaint: pain in the front of the knee.
Treatment: decrease intensity of training.
Surgery: not necessary.
- **Ankle sprain**—acute injury.
Cause: landing improperly.
Presenting complaint: pain on the outside of the ankle.
Treatment: x-ray to rule out a fracture, immobilization.
Surgery: rarely necessary.
- **Severs syndrome**—overuse injury.
Cause: running and jumping.
Presenting complaint: pain in the back of the heel.
Treatment: decrease in training activity.
Surgery: not necessary.

YOUNG BALLERINAS CAN SUSTAIN OVERUSE INJURIES TO THE LOWER EXTREMITIES.

FOOTBALL, RUGBY, SOCCER, AND LACROSSE

These are immensely popular sports in the United States. In football alone there are over one million injuries to adolescents each year. Common football, rugby, soccer, and lacrosse injuries are:

- **Burners**—acute injury.
Cause: either traction or compression of the nerves leading from the neck to the arm from a blow to the head or shoulder.
Presenting complaint: burning pain down the arm, weakness.
Treatment: withholding from competition until symptoms resolve, extra padding.
Surgery: not necessary.

- **Anterior shoulder dislocation**—acute but can be recurrent with little provocation after the initial injury.
  Cause: forcibly pushing the outstretched arm backwards and away from the body.
  Presenting complaint: shoulder pain, lack of mobility.
  Treatment: reduction of dislocation followed by rehabilitation exercises.
  Surgery: necessary for recurrent dislocations.
- **Hip pointer**—acute injury.
  Cause: blow to the side of the hip.
  Presenting complaint: hip pain.
  Treatment: properly fitting hip pads, R.I.C.E.
  Surgery: not necessary.
- **Groin muscle strain**—acute injury.
  Cause: colliding with another player while kicking the ball.
  Presenting complaint: pain and swelling on the inside of the thigh.
  Treatment: refraining from competition until symptoms resolve, R.I.C.E.
  Surgery: not necessary.
- **Quadriceps contusion**—acute injury.
  Cause: player struck in the leg by another player.
  Presenting complaint: pain in the anterior thigh.
  Treatment: splinting the leg in a bent position, properly fitting thigh pads, R.I.C.E.
  Surgery: not necessary.
- **Ankle sprain**—acute injury.
  Cause: landing improperly (very common in soccer).
  Presenting complaint: pain on the outside of the ankle.
  Treatment: X-ray to rule out a fracture, R.I.C.E., immobilization.
  Surgery: rarely necessary.
- **Turf toe**—acute and recurrent injury.
  Cause: forcibly pushing off of the big toe, especially on rigid surfaces such as artificial turf.
  Presenting complaint: pain at the base of the big toe, especially when pushing off.
  Treatment: strapping and taping.
  Surgery: not necessary.

! Tips for coaches.

Prevention: *Make sure that your players are properly equipped with well-fitting helmets. Most youth players wear helmets with an inflatable liner. Check each player's helmet personally. Don't relegate this task to one of the parents. Make sure that each player wears a mouthpiece at all times. If a player complains of headache, dizziness, or is confused, keep him out of practice and competition until he is cleared to play by a doctor. Instruct your players in proper tackling technique. Encourage resistance training, which strengthens the neck. Teach your players to "wrap up" when making a tackle to prevent shoulder dislocations.*

Treatment: If you think that a player has sustained a serious injury, call 911 and check for the ABCs: airway, breathing, circulation. Never move an unconscious player or one who complains of neck pain.

GYMNASTICS AND CHEERLEADING

Gymnasts and cheerleaders can sustain the same types of strains and sprains that affect other athletes. Their most common significant injury is the ankle sprain, but they can also suffer both acute and overuse injuries of the upper as well as the lower extremities because they bear their entire body weight on their hands and arms during certain events. Cheerleaders who are at the bottom of pyramids or who support a partner during stunts have an increased incidence of upper extremity overuse injury. Gymnasts have a high incidence of stress fractures of the lumbar spine because of performing many maneuvers with their backs arched (hyperextended). This is particularly true during the dismount phase of the gymnasts' routine, which requires landing with great force with the back arched. They share this problem, called spondylolisthesis (for the explanation see the section on back injuries), particularly with football linemen and divers.

GYMNASTS' MOST COMMON SIGNIFICANT INJURY IS THE ANKLE SPRAIN.

In gymnastics, boys compete on the pommel horse, vault, rings, floor exercise, and parallel and horizontal bars. Girls' competition includes floor exercises, vault, uneven parallel bars, and the balance beam. Male gymnasts can experience more upper body injuries than females because of the difference in events in which they compete. Notwithstanding this fact, the majority of injuries to both boys and girls involve the lower extremities.

Female gymnasts are also at high risk for what we call the *female athlete triad,* which includes thin body type, eating disorders, and no menstrual periods. This situation predisposes them to osteoporosis. There is currently a move afoot in international gymnastics to change the way events are judged, so that the underdeveloped, young female body type is not rated as highly as it has been in the past.

Another problem that places both gymnasts and cheerleaders at increased risk of injury is that these athletes compete year-round, which increases the risk of both overuse injuries and acute injuries due to fatigue.

Common gymnastic and cheerleading injuries are:

- **Wrist sprain**—acute injury.
  Cause: landing improperly.
  Presenting complaint: wrist pain usually on the thumb side of the wrist.
  Treatment: x-ray to rule out a fracture, avoiding practice until pain resolves, R.I.C.E.
  Surgery: not necessary.
- **Wrist fracture**—can be acute or overuse (stress fracture of the growth plate).
  Cause: fall (acute), repetitive weight bearing on the hands (overuse).
  Presenting complaint: wrist pain.
  Treatment: immobilization in a cast, reduction if displaced.
  Surgery: sometimes necessary, particularly of nonunion, when the fracture fragments won't knit.
- **Ankle sprain**—acute injury.
  Cause: landing improperly.
  Presenting complaint: pain on the outside of the ankle.
  Treatment: X-ray to rule out a fracture, R.I.C.E., immobilization.
  Surgery: rarely necessary.

Lacerations are common in hockey as a result of a blow by the puck or stick or from the skate blade. Facial lacerations were exceedingly common in the past, but with the rule requiring helmets, the incidences have been greatly reduced. Facial lacerations and eye injuries can be further reduced when face masks similar to those worn by football players are attached to the helmets. The ice hockey helmet is anchored at only two points, which many sports medicine experts believe is responsible for lacerations to the chin and bridge of the nose when the helmet slides up and down. They suggest a four-point fixation system like that used for helmets in football and lacrosse, to further reduce these injuries. If lacerations do occur, they can be sutured or treated with superglue so that the athlete can return to play without subjecting other participants to risk from bloodborne diseases. Because ice hockey is a collision sport, head and neck injuries can also occur frequently. Other common injuries are:

- **Shoulder separations**—acute injury.
  Cause: direct blow to the shoulder.
  Presenting complaint: shoulder pain, especially in motion.
  Treatment: refraining from competition if pain is severe, extra padding.
  Surgery: only necessary for third-degree sprains and then mostly cosmetic.
- **Collarbone fractures**—acute injury.
  Cause: direct blow to the shoulder.
  Presenting complaint: pain, usually in the middle of the collarbone, worse with motion of the shoulder, bump at fracture site.
  Treatment: figure-of-eight splint.
  Surgery: only for fractures in an unusual location.

! Tips for coaches

Prevention: helmets with four-point fixation.

ICE SKATING AND ROLLERBLADING

The novice ice skater or rollerblader can sustain acute injuries as a result of falls. Rollerbladers should wear protective helmets as well as knee, wrist, and elbow pads. They should also wear long slacks to prevent abrasions when they fall and slide on the pavement. Other common skating injuries are:

- **Wrist fractures**—acute injury.
  Cause: falling on the outstretched hand.
  Presenting complaint: wrist pain, bump on the top of the wrist.
  Treatment: immobilization in a cast.
  Surgery: occasionally necessary.
- **Jumper's knee**—overuse injury.
  Cause: repeated jumping.
  Presenting complaint: pain in the front of the knee.
  Treatment: decrease in intensity of training, R.I.C.E.
  Surgery: not necessary.

SKIING

Almost a half million skiing injuries occur in the United States each year. Because of improved equipment, this represents a lower rate of injury than was experienced a couple of decades ago. Downhill skiers suffer traumatic injuries almost exclusively; they rarely suffer overuse injuries. Most injuries occur in the later part of the morning and afternoon skiing sessions, which suggests that fatigue is a factor.

AN INJURY UNIQUE TO DOWNHILL SKIING IS THE BOOT TOP FRACTURE.

Most skiing injuries involve the leg, although improved boots and bindings have dramatically reduced the incidence of this type of injury. An injury unique to downhill skiing is the *boot top fracture,* even though improved equipment has greatly lessened lower leg and ankle injury. The injury occurs when the boot bindings do not release and the skier falls, fracturing the tibia and fibula at the level of the boot top.

Another common injury occurs when a skier falls and the thumb gets caught in the ski pole tether. This thumb injury is discussed in greater detail in part 3 in the section dealing with hand injuries.

Because downhill skiers can go as fast as automobiles, a collision with a tree or another skier can result in death. The majority of these deaths occur in males between the ages of fifteen and twenty-four as a result of risk-taking behavior, and the accidents often involve alcohol.

Cross-country skiers, on the other hand, experience an estimated 75 percent of overuse injuries. Traumatic injuries in both sports usually involve the lower extremities and occur while the skier is going downhill. Other common skiing injuries are:

- **Concussion**—acute injury.
  Cause: direct blow to the head (e.g., falling striking a tree).
  Presenting complaint: confusion, loss of consciousness.
  Treatment: If the skier is unconscious, don't move him or her. Call the ski patrol.
  Surgery: not necessary.
- **Knee sprains**—acute injury.
  Cause: twisting the body with the ski planted.
  Presenting complaint: knee pain, swelling.
  Treatment: avoiding skiing, R.I.C.E.
  Surgery: often necessary in third-degree anterior cruciate ligament sprains.
- **Achilles tendinitis**—overuse injury.
  Cause: repeated striding.
  Presenting complaint: pain in the back of the heel.
  Treatment: avoiding skiing, modifying technique, R.I.C.E.
  Surgery: sometimes necessary for a ruptured tendon.
- **Turf toe**—acute and recurrent injury.
  Cause: forcibly pushing off from the big toe.
  Presenting complaint: pain at the base of the big toe, especially when pushing off.
  Treatment: strapping and taping.
  Surgery: not necessary.

Shoulder injuries are very common among competitive swimmers, who average about half a million strokes during a season. One study suggested that 90 percent of swimmers will experience shoulder problems at some time during their careers. Most of these injuries are either rotator cuff *tendinitis* or *bursitis.* The incidence of these injuries can be decreased by proper training technique. I advise against using paddles, which increase the strain on the shoulder, and kickboards, which cause the rotator cuff to be pinched under one of the shoulder bones while the arms are extended in front of the swimmer.

Most coaches limit the use of different strokes in practice. They have swimmers practice the freestyle stroke at least 50 percent of the time, regardless of what stroke the athlete uses in competition, because the freestyle stroke is easier on the shoulder. Practice is primarily about building endurance, not about perfecting technique.

SWIMMER'S EAR IS A BACTERIAL INFECTION CAUSED BY MICROORGANISMS IN THE POOL WATER.

Swimmer's ear is a bacterial infection caused by microorganisms in the pool water. Ordinary earplugs are not effective in preventing swimmer's ear, and custom earplugs are expensive. I recommend that swimmers either use Silly Putty as an earplug or put two drops of a mixture of equal parts vinegar and rubbing alcohol into the ear after coming out of the pool for the day. This will reduce the incidence of infection. The Silly Putty earplugs are particularly useful in swimmers who have had pressure-equalizing tubes surgically implanted in their ears. If, despite these precautions, your child develops an ear infection, your physician can prescribe antibiotic eardrops to cure it.

Swimmers also get a chemical *conjunctivitis* from the chlorine in the pool. This is a type of pinkeye caused by a chemical rather than an infectious agent. Many swimmers wear goggles to prevent this condition. It can be treated with Acular prescription eyedrops.

Many asthmatics choose swimming as their sport because they are habitually breathing warm humidified air just above the pool's surface. This air is much less likely to precipitate an asthmatic attack than the cold, dry air inhaled by cross-country skiers. Exercise-induced asthma can occur and should be treated as outlined in the section on chest problems. Other common swimming injuries are:

- **Patello-femoral stress syndrome**—overuse injury.
  Cause: breast-stroke kick, particularly in women.
  Presenting complaint: pain in the front of the knee.
  Treatment: decrease in training intensity, R.I.C.E., change to another stroke, quadriceps-strengthening exercises.
  Surgery: not necessary.
- **Spondylolysis and spondylolisthesis**—overuse injury.
  Cause: repeated arching of the back, especially associated with breast stroke.
  Presenting complaint: low back pain.
  Treatment: change in strokes, bracing.
  Surgery: rarely necessary.

! Tips for coaches.

Prevention: *Use Silly Putty earplugs.*
Treatment: Use rubbing alcohol and vinegar for swimmer's ear.

TENNIS AND OTHER RACQUET SPORTS

Squash and racquetball are played in confined spaces where the ball or racquet is likely to strike an opponent. This is a cause of both lacerations and contusions. The incidence of eye injuries can be decreased dramatically by wearing protective goggles, which is imperative in these sports. *Tennis elbow* is an inflammation of the tendon of the muscles that flex the wrist. The condition occurs because of poor technique when hitting the backhand stroke (see the discussion of elbow injuries in part 3). Other tennis and racket sports injuries are:

THE INCIDENCE OF EYE INJURIES CAN BE DECREASED DRAMATICALLY BY WEARING PROTECTIVE GOGGLES.

- **Rotator cuff tendinitis**—overuse injury.

  Cause: serving.

  Presenting complaint: shoulder pain with repeated overhand strokes.

  Treatment: decreased training intensity, R.I.C.E., muscle-strengthening exercises.

  Surgery: necessary only in case of rotator cuff tears, which are rare among young athletes.

- **Ankle sprain**—acute injury.

  Cause: landing improperly.

  Presenting complaint: pain on the outside of the ankle.

  Treatment: X-ray to rule out a fracture, R.I.C.E., immobilization.

  Surgery: rarely necessary.

WRESTLING

We should not be surprised that the incidence of injuries in wrestling is about the same as in other collision sports, such as football, ice hockey, and lacrosse. It should also not be surprising that younger participants are injured less frequently than their older counterparts. The younger athletes have less muscle mass and therefore create less force with each maneuver.

Injuries occur as a result of direct contact with an opponent: falling, twisting, and friction with an opponent or the mat. Wrestlers are also subject to overuse injuries from overtraining.

Wrestlers sustain a relatively large number of facial lacerations because, unlike players in other collision sports, they do not wear helmets. This fact leads to another type of injury peculiar to wrestling and boxing, the *cauliflower ear.* This injury can be prevented with well-fitting protective headgear.

Wrestlers suffer a large number of *skin infections* as a result of close contact, lack of protective equipment, and the warm, moist environment in which the sport is conducted. Both *bacterial* and *viral* infections are transmitted. A herpes infection, *herpes gladiatorum,* is so named because of its association with the sport. If the child has a skin infection, he or she should be withheld from competition. In fact, the NCAA won't let a wrestler compete who has had a recent herpes infection until he or she is free of new lesions for three days and is taking Acyclovir, an anti-viral agent. Wrestling mats should be cleaned regularly with an antiseptic solution (a weak solution of chlorine bleach).

Another problem that we see in wrestling is *weight fluctuations*. Repeated, sudden drops in weight are common; one sports medicine expert estimated that one-third of wrestlers lose between one and ten pounds a hundred times in their wrestling career! Wrestlers "make weight" by a combination of not eating and dehydrating themselves. Both of these practices can be harmful and should be discouraged by physicians and coaches. All youth wrestlers and many youth football players have to lose weight at some time in their career to compete in a certain weight class. It is difficult to generalize when giving advice to parents regarding how much weight an athlete can safely lose and over what period of time this feat should be accomplished. A child who is overweight with a 25 percent body fat composition can easily lose 20 pounds over a several-month period to compete at the 180-pound weight class. A lean thirteen-year-old with a 5 percent fat composition should not try to lose 10 pounds so that he can play for the 110-pound football team rather than the 125-pound team. Football players have to "make weight" only once each season. They usually have a weigh-in several days before their first game. Wrestlers have to "make weight" before each match and they typically have to wrestle soon after the weigh-in. Therefore, a football player would be at less risk for dehydration and injury than a wrestler if he skipped a meal or two and exercised vigorously to sweat off that last pound before weighing in.

A HERPES INFECTION, HERPES GLADIATORUM, IS SO NAMED BECAUSE OF ITS ASSOCIATION WITH THE SPORT.

Adolescent boys should have a body fat composition of approximately 7 percent. Sports medicine physicians can measure body fat percentages by measuring skin-fold thickness to determine how much weight a wrestler should lose and advise him at what weight class to compete. Wisconsin recently adopted mandatory rules regarding the appropriate weight class at which each wrestler should compete. These rules are based on skin-fold measurements done by experienced testers using calipers (a sort of sophisticated "pinch an inch" measurement). Other common wrestling injuries are:

- **Neck sprain**—acute injury.
  Cause: take downs, half nelson.
  Presenting complaint: neck pain.
  Treatment: avoiding training and competition.
  Surgery: not necessary.
- **Anterior shoulder dislocation**—acute but can be recurrent with little provocation after the initial injury.
  Cause: forcibly pushing the outstretched arm backwards and away from the body.
  Presenting complaint: shoulder pain, lack of mobility.
  Treatment: reduction of the dislocation followed by rehabilitation exercises.
- **Knee sprains**—acute injury.
  Cause: twisting the body with the foot planted.
  Presenting complaint: knee pain, swelling.
  Treatment: avoidance of competition until symptoms abate, R.I.C.E.
  Surgery: often necessary in third-degree anterior cruciate ligament sprains.

FIVE

The

Medical

Bag

spend a significant part of my medical practice teaching medical students. One day I was expounding to a medical student on one or another theory pertaining to sports medicine when she asked me, "What do you carry in your medical bag when you attend a sporting event as a team physician?" The question stopped me in my tracks: I simply carried whatever happened to be in the medical bag since I had last looked at it. I realized that it wouldn't be very satisfying to tell her that so I told her what I think *should* be in a sports medicine physician's medical bag. Some parents may also be physicians and may agree at some point to serve as team doctor. If you have not played this role before, you may not have a clear idea about what medical equipment is most suitable to bring to a game. The following is a list of the basics:

- Fluorescein dye to test for corneal abrasions
- Irrigating solution (salt water) for rinsing foreign material out of the eye
- Eye patches to patch the eye in case of corneal abrasions
- An otoscope and ophthalmoscope (medical instruments for examining the eyes and ears)
- Alkali solution, to be used in place of milk, for rinsing a lost tooth prior to reimplantation
- Suture material, scissors, and a needle holder to repair lacerations, or a tube of superglue
- Inhaled bronchodilator to treat asthmatics (e.g., Proventil)
- Injectable adrenaline for asthma and insect stings in susceptible patients
- A stethoscope and a blood pressure cuff (at football games I also bring a large cuff for the large athletes)
- A tube of cake icing to give to diabetics who are having an insulin reaction
  In addition to these items, there are other provisions that should be on hand but are generally too big to fit in the medical bag. These include:
- Bolt cutters or a battery-operated screwdriver to remove the helmet of an injured athlete
- A knee immobilizer (one of those long white things with Velcro closures to keep the knee straight)
- A splint to keep the arm straight
- A portable phone to call 911 when necessary
    The trainer should also have ice, tape, ace bandages, scissors, etc., on hand, which are indispensable at sporting events.

THE TEN COMMANDMENTS FOR PARENTS OF YOUNG ATHLETES

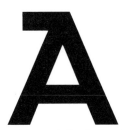

As I stand on the sidelines or sit in the bleachers at various sporting events, I'm often asked my advice on various sports-related topics. Many parents know that I have a large family of pretty good athletes, so they expect me to have some ideas that might help them cope with the tribulations of raising young athletes. The following stories illustrate some insights that I have gleaned over the years.

I was playing shortstop in a father-son baseball game next to a third baseman who had known me since college. I backhanded a ball in the hole at short and threw the ball to first base on about six hops. I turned to my friend and said, "I must be getting old. I can't make that throw anymore." He looked at me and said, "You couldn't make that throw when you were twenty years old." My friend was right! We tend to look at our children through adult eyes. We expect them to do what we would do if we were playing our best. This is complicated by the fact that most of us are guilty of having a selective memory. I recently saw a bumper sticker at a track meet that said, "The older I get the faster I was." **The First Commandment: Enjoy watching your children play at their level, and be patient and understanding. They're probably about as good as you were at their age.**

I've been around youth sports for twenty years, and I'm a pretty good judge of talent. I am certainly wise enough to know that my daughter should be the starting point guard on her basketball team. **The Second Commandment: The best coaches are the ones who are smart enough to realize that your child has talent. These coaches start your children, usually at the most important skill position.**

One of my sons was a very good high school football player. He had a distinguished high school career and was voted to the all-conference team. He attended a division one college, where in four years he saw very little playing time. His biggest contribution was on the scout team, but he kept on playing when others quit because he loved the game. His coaches always respected this enthusiasm and his contribution to the team. **The Third Commandment: The truly best coaches are the ones who, despite the fact that they don't play your child, understand that all the players on a team make a contribution to the team's effort. They treat all players with respect regardless of their ability.**

I coached a youth basketball team on which one of my sons played. At the sports banquet at the end of the season, all the teams fielded by my children's school got together for an awards presentation. All the other coaches presented their entire teams with eight-inch-tall trophies for participating on the various teams. Most of these teams had a losing record during the season. My team, which had some excellent athletes, finished third in the A division, but I gave trophies only to the most valuable and the most improved players (my son didn't win either of these awards). I did not give participation awards to any of my players. Some of the parents were upset with me for not awarding trophies for participation. **The Fourth Commandment: There is a difference between winning and losing. There is no shame in losing if we do our best. But it's still not winning. One of the lessons that sport teaches is to win with grace and lose with dignity but to know the difference between the two. Don't blur the distinction.**

My son, a senior in high school, helped me coach my daughter's basketball team one season. He was shocked by the fact that parents made negative comments about their daughters' skills. They were outspokenly critical of mistakes that the girls made. Your child isn't likely to be paid to play professional sports. Only 3 percent of high school basketball players play basketball in college and only 1 percent of them play in the pros. **The Fifth Commandment: Be positive and proud. Your children are having fun and learning. It's a game. Appreciate it for what it is.**

6 It's not only your children who don't get paid to play sports; the coaches are volunteers, and the officials either are volunteers or are paid a nominal amount for their efforts. Often they are learning too. **The Sixth Commandment: Go easy on coaches and officials. Whatever game your child is playing, it's probably not the seventh game of the World Series.**

7 From my years of experience as a coach, I have learned that kids need both positive and negative instructions in sports, as in every other aspect of their life. Sometimes they need a pat on the back; sometimes they need to be yelled at. You have to know when to do which. **The Seventh Commandment: When you're correcting your children, be positive about 90 percent of the time and negative 10 percent of the time.**

8 Over the years I've seen too many coaches and parents harangue a child immediately after he or she made the mistake that caused the child's team to lose the game. Never be negative immediately after your child makes a costly mistake. If your daughter let the ground ball go through her legs and thus allowed the game-winning run to score, it is not the time to tell her to look the ball into the glove. She realizes it! **The Eighth Commandment: If you wish to criticize technique, don't do it after your child has made a costly mistake. Wait until the sting of the moment has cooled so that your comments sound like constructive criticism, not blame.**

I was standing on the sidelines next to the coach at a high school conference championship football game. It was late in the fourth quarter and the score was tied. The other team had to punt from deep in their own territory. One of our best players was the punt returner. He dropped the punt and the other team recovered. We stopped their drive and they had to punt again. The same player dropped another punt and the opposition again recovered. By this time the punt returner was on the brink of tears as he walked off the field. The coach went over to the player, but instead of berating him for making a critical mistake *twice*, he said, "You are a good player. Don't worry; you won't drop another punt for the rest of the year." What a confidence builder! We held the other team and got the ball back, finally winning the game. Our punt returner was also a receiver who caught a key pass in our winning drive. **The Ninth Commandment: These kids have fragile egos and they depend on their parents and coaches for validation of their self-worth. When they're down, say something to pick them up.**

Parents frequently want to know when their children can start playing a sport. They are often first-time parents who are filled with exuberance about their children competing in organized sports for the first time. I don't want to be a curmudgeon and dampen their enthusiasm, but I'd like to offer the following reflection. The day may come when your son or daughter wants to quit a sport. You may see your daughter as the next Mary Lou Retton, but she has grown tired of practicing four hours a day, six days a week. Her heart is set on running for class president or starring on the debate team. Though you may not see it, she knows that she is a mediocre gymnast with no hope of participating at the next level. **The Tenth Commandment: Parents, don't live vicariously through your children. Encourage them in their sports but don't force them to participate. It's more important to know when your child's sports career should end than when it should begin.**

GLOSSARY

Many of the concepts in sports medicine are simple and straightforward; only the terminology is difficult. The following terms and definitions are commonly used.

abrasion—Scrape.

acute vs. chronic—Immediate vs. long-standing. An acute injury is one that is less than two weeks' duration. A chronic injury has been symptomatic for more than six weeks. Any injury of intermediate duration is considered subacute.

aerobic—Pertaining to activity that can be performed without building up an oxygen debt. In other words, an aerobic activity is one that we can perform while carrying on a conversation, or that produces a heart rate that is at 75 percent of our predicted maximum heart rate. These activities include brisk walking, jogging, ice skating, bicycling, swimming, and rowing.

amnesia—Impairment of memory.

anaerobic—Pertaining to activity in which we build up an oxygen debt. In other words, anaerobic activity is one that causes us to huff and puff while we are performing it. These activities involve sudden bursts of activity, such as sprinting.

anterior and posterior—Front and back. The anterior compartment is in the front of the leg. The posterior compartment is in the back of the leg.

asymptomatic—Not causing any symptoms.

avulse—Tear off. In an avulsion fracture, a piece of bone is sheared off the main segment of bone.

cardiovascular system—The system of the body composed of the heart and blood vessels.

chronic—See **acute vs. chronic**.

comminuted fracture—A fracture in which the bone is shattered in several pieces.

compound fracture—A fracture in which part of the bone protrudes through the skin. Also known as an **open fracture**.

concussion—An interruption of normal brain function without any anatomic change.

contusion—Bruise.

CT scan or CAT—Computerized tomography or computerized axial tomography. A medical imaging technique using x-rays and a computer to create a picture.

displaced—Out of place. The term refers to fractures in which the two segments of the fractured bone are not lined up with each other.

distal—See **proximal and distal**.

dorsal and ventral—Top and bottom. The dorsal aspect of the hand is the top of the hand when it is prone on a table.

echocardiogram—A diagnostic test that employs ultrasound waves to make a picture of the heart.

extend—Straighten, lengthen the muscle.

evert—Twist outward.

flex—Bend, contract the muscle.

fractured—Broken. Parents often ask, "Is it fractured or broken?" These terms mean exactly the same thing.

femur—The long bone in the thigh.

fibula—The smaller, long bone in the lower leg. It is the bone on the outside of the leg at the ankle.

heart murmur—A whooshing sound heard with a stethoscope when a physician listens to the heart. It is caused by turbulent blood flow.

humerus—Long bone in the upper arm.

hyper and hypo—High and low, or over and under. Hyperthyroidism refers to an overactive thyroid gland. Hypoglycemia is low blood sugar.

inhaled bronchodilators—Inhaled medications that relax spasms of the muscles lining the small airways of the lungs. They are used to treat wheezing.

invert—Twist inward.

laceration—Cut.

ligament—A band of fibrous tissue connecting one bone to another.

lower extremity—The leg.

medial and lateral—Inside and outside. The medial collateral ligament of the knee is on the inside of the knee joint, and the lateral collateral ligament is on the outside of the knee joint.

menstrual cycle—The time from the first day of a woman's period until the day before the first day of her next period.

MRI–Magnetic resonance imaging. It is medical imaging technique that utilizes the principle that different tissues vibrate differently when exposed to a magnet. A computer can calculate these differences and create an image.

nondisplaced—Aligned. Refers to fractures in which the two segments of bone are in good alignment.

nonunion—Refers to a fracture that won't knit. The fracture fragments are usually in good alignment but won't heal.

palpate—Feel.

posterior—*See* **anterior and posterior**.

proximal and distal—Near and far. The proximal part of the bone is nearest the center of the body; the distal part is farthest from the center of the body.

puberty—The age of sexual maturity. In both boys and girls, the time when the reproductive organs have reached adult size and functional ability. In males it is easier to determine because the organs are external. In females we use the onset of regular menstrual periods as a sign.

radius—Larger of the long bones in the forearm. It is on the side of the thumb at the wrist.

simple fracture—A fracture in which the overlying skin is intact. Also called a **closed fracture**.

sprain—An overstretched ligament. Sprains are graded first-degree through third-degree. In a first-degree sprain there is no interruption of the integrity of the ligament. A second-degree sprain involves some tearing and loss of strength of the ligament. A third-degree sprain is a complete rupture of the structure.

strain—An overstretched muscle. Strains are graded first-degree through third-degree. In a first-degree strain there is no loss of strength and no disruption of the muscle fibers. In a second-degree strain there is loss of strength and less than a 50 percent disruption of the muscle fiber. In a third-degree strain the muscle is completely torn.

tendon—The end of a muscle where it tapers, becomes fibrous, and attaches itself to the bone.

tibia—The larger of the two long bones in the lower leg below the knee. It is the bone on the inside of the leg at the ankle.

ulna—The smaller long bone in the forearm below the elbow. It is on the side of the little finger at the wrist.

ultrasound—A diagnostic imaging study utilizing sound waves to make a picture of internal organs.

upper extremity—The arm.

ventral—*See* **dorsal and ventral**.

Date

Name   Sex   Age   Date of Birth

Grade   Sport(s)

Personal physician   Address   Physician's phone

EXPLAIN "YES" ANSWERS BELOW: Yes   No

1. Have you ever been hospitalized? .... ☐ ☐
   Have you ever had surgery? .... ☐ ☐
2. Are you presently taking any medications or pills? .... ☐ ☐
3. Do you have any allergies (medicine, bees or other stinging insects)? .... ☐ ☐
4. Have you ever passed out during or after exercise? .... ☐ ☐
   Have you ever been dizzy during or after exercise? .... ☐ ☐
   Have you ever had chest pain during or after exercise? .... ☐ ☐
   Do you tire more quickly than your friends during exercise? .... ☐ ☐
   Have you ever had high blood pressure? .... ☐ ☐
   Have you ever been told that you have a heart murmur? .... ☐ ☐
   Have you ever had racing of your heart or skipped heartbeats? .... ☐ ☐
   Has anyone in your family died of heart problems
     or a sudden death before age 50? .... ☐ ☐
5. Do you have any skin problems (itching, rashes, acne)? .... ☐ ☐
6. Have you ever had a head injury? .... ☐ ☐
   Have you ever been knocked out or unconscious? .... ☐ ☐
   Have you ever had a seizure? .... ☐ ☐
   Have you ever had a stinger, burner, or pinched nerve? .... ☐ ☐
7. Have you ever had heat or muscle cramps? .... ☐ ☐
   Have you ever been dizzy or passed out in the heat? .... ☐ ☐
8. Do you have trouble breathing or do you cough during or after activity? .... ☐ ☐
9. Do you use any special equipment (pads, braces,
   neck rolls, mouth guard, eye guards, etc.)? .... ☐ ☐
10. Have you had any problems with your eyes or vision? .... ☐ ☐
    Do you wear glasses or contacts or protective eye wear? .... ☐ ☐
11. Have you ever sprained/strained, dislocated, fractured, broken,
    or had repeated swelling or other injuries of any bones or joints? .... ☐ ☐
    ☐ Head   ☐ Shoulder   ☐ Thigh   ☐ Neck   ☐ Elbow   ☐ Knee   ☐ Chest
    ☐ Forearm   ☐ Shin/calf   ☐ Back   ☐ Wrist   ☐ Ankle   ☐ Hip   ☐ Hand   ☐ Foot
12. Have you had any other medical problems
    (infectious mononucleosis, diabetes, etc.)? .... ☐ ☐
13. Have you had a medical problem or injury since your last evaluation? .... ☐ ☐
14. When was your last tetanus shot? .... ☐ ☐
    When was your last measles immunization? .... ☐ ☐
15. When was your first menstrual period? .... ☐ ☐
    When was your last menstrual period? .... ☐ ☐
    What was the longest time between your periods last year? .... ☐ ☐

Explain "Yes" answers: ....
....

I hereby state that, to the best of my knowledge, my answers to the above questions are correct.

Signature of athlete   Date

Signature of parent/guardian

Date _____

Name _____ Age _____ Date of Birth _____

Height _____ Weight _____ BP _____ Pulse _____

Vision R20/ _____ L20/ _____ Corrected: Y _____ N _____ Pupils _____

	NORMAL	ABNORMAL FINDINGS				INITIALS
Cardiopulmonary						
Pulses						
Heart						
Lungs						
Tannner stage	1	2	3	4	5	
Skin						
Abdominal						
Genitalia						
Musculoskeletal						
Neck						
Shoulder						
Elbow						
Wrist						
Hand						
Back						
Knee						
Ankle						
Foot						
Other						

Clearance:

     A. Cleared

     B. Cleared after completing evaluation/rehabilitation for: _____

     C. Not cleared for: ☐ Collision

                   ☐ Contact

                   ☐ Noncontact ____Strenuous ____Moderately strenuous ____Nonstrenuous

Due to: ....

Recommendation: ....

....

....

Name of physician: ....Date ....

Address: ....Phone ....

Signature of physician: ....

Preparticipation physical evaluation (monograph). Kansas City, MO: American Academy of Family Physicians, American Academy of Pediatrics, American Medical Society for Sports Medicine, American Orthopaedic Society for Sports Medicine, American Osteopathic Academy of Sports Medicine, 1992.

INDEX

SPORTS MEDICINE FOR PARENTS & COACHES

Posterior cruciate ligaments, 64–65, **65**
Posterior shoulder dislocation, 42–43
Pregame meals, 27
Pregame warm-ups, 18–20
Preparticipation physical exams, 7–9
Preschoolers, 2–3
Preseason training, 15
Pressure-equalizing tubes, 40, 97
Primary care sports medicine physicians, 23
Pronation, 70, **76**
Proprioception, 73
Protective cups, 58–59
Protective goggles, 9, 38–39
Proventil, 56, 103
Pseudoanemia, 22–23
Puberty, 4–5
Pump bumps, 75
Punch-drunk syndrome, 87

Q
Quadriceps, 63–64, **64**
Quadriceps contusion, 64, **64**, 91
Quadriplegic athletes, 11–12

R
Racquetball injuries, 98–99
Range of motion, 31
Recurrent sprains, 73
Rehabilitation, 32–33
Reinforcement, positive, 106–107
Reinjury, 30
Resistance training, 92
Respect, 105
Respiratory problems, 56–57
Rest, relative, 39
Retin-A, 79
Retina, detached, 93
Retton, Mary Lou, 107
Reye's syndrome, 32

R.I.C.E. treatment, 31–32, 55, 68, 83
Ritalin, 13
Rollerblading injuries, 95
Rotator cuffs
  tears, 84
  tendinitis, 101
Rugby injuries, 90–92
Runners, 21–22
  injuries, 66–69, 88
  shoes, 88–89
Ruptures
  Achilles tendon, 86
  anterior cruciate ligament, 64, **65**
  bladder, 11–12
  spleen, 10, 57
  testicle, 58–59

S
Salt tablets, 18
Salt water, 103
Scaphoid navicular (wrist bone) fractures, 50–51
Scheuermann's disease, 61, **61**
Scissors, 103
Screwdriver, battery-operated, 103
Second impact syndrome, 35
Seizures, 10
Self-worth, 107
Semilunar cartilage, 66
Severs syndrome, 74–75, **74**, 90
Shin splints, 70
Shock pads, 37
Shoes, 76–77, 88
Shoulders
  dislocation, 41–43, **42**
  injuries, 41–46
  Little League, 44, **45**
  musculature instability, 44, 46
  separation sprain, 43, **43**, 94
  socket, 41, **41**
  strap, figure-of-eight, 44, **44**
  stress fracture, 44, **44**

Sickle-cell disease/anemia, 23
Sickle-cell trait, 22–23
Silly putty, 39–40, 97–98
Sinus infections, 40
Six-to nine-year-olds, 3–4
Skier's thumb, 52–53, **53**
Skiing injuries, 95–96
Skin-fold measurements, 100
Skin
  infections, 80–81, 99
  injuries, 77–80
Slipped capital femoral epiphysis disruption, 62, **62**
Soccer injuries, 57, 90–92
Sockets
  hip, **41**
  shoulder, **41**
Socks, 79
Spearing, 36
Spenco longitudinal arch supports, 76
Spinal canals, 36
Spine, stress fractures of, 60, **60**
Spleens, 10, 57
Splints, 103
Spondylolisthesis, 60–61
Spondylolysis, 60–61, **60**
Sports
  physically appropriate, 5–7
Sports bras, 10
Sports drinks, 18, 72
Sports goggles, 38
Sports-specific exercises, 18
Sprains, 29
  ankle, 73–74, **73–74**
  ligament, 43, 73–74, **73–74**
  recurrent, 73
  separation, 43–44, **43**, 94
  wrist, 51, 93
Squash injuries, 98–99
Static stretching, 18–19
Station exams, 8
Steroids, anabolic, 24
Stethoscopes, 103
Stinger, 36–37